W9-CML-638

THE MARKEY SCHOLARS CONFERENCE

PROCEEDINGS

George R. Reinhart, Editor

Committee for the Evaluation of the
Lucille P. Markey Programs in Biomedical Sciences

Board on Higher Education and Workforce

Policy and Global Affairs Division

NATIONAL RESEARCH COUNCIL
OF THE NATIONAL ACADEMIES

THE NATIONAL ACADEMIES PRESS
Washington, D.C.
www.nap.edu

THE NATIONAL ACADEMIES PRESS 500 Fifth Street, N.W. Washington, DC 20001

NOTICE: The project that is the subject of this report was approved by the Governing Board of the National Research Council, whose members are drawn from the councils of the National Academy of Sciences, the National Academy of Engineering, and the Institute of Medicine. The members of the committee responsible for the report were chosen for their special competences and with regard for appropriate balance.

This project was supported by Grant No. 98-1 between the Lucille P. Markey Charitable Trust and the National Academy of Sciences. Any opinions, findings, conclusions, or recommendations expressed in this publication are those of the author(s) and do not necessarily reflect the views of the organizations or agencies that provided support for the project.

International Standard Book Number 0-309-09173-X (Book)
International Standard Book Number 0-309-53101-2 (PDF)

Additional copies of this report are available from the National Academies Press, 500 Fifth Street, N.W., Lockbox 285, Washington, DC 20055; (800) 624-6242 or (202) 334-3313 (in the Washington metropolitan area); Internet, http://www.nap.edu

THE NATIONAL ACADEMIES
Advisers to the Nation on Science, Engineering, and Medicine

The **National Academy of Sciences** is a private, nonprofit, self-perpetuating society of distinguished scholars engaged in scientific and engineering research, dedicated to the furtherance of science and technology and to their use for the general welfare. Upon the authority of the charter granted to it by the Congress in 1863, the Academy has a mandate that requires it to advise the federal government on scientific and technical matters. Dr. Bruce M. Alberts is president of the National Academy of Sciences.

The **National Academy of Engineering** was established in 1964, under the charter of the National Academy of Sciences, as a parallel organization of outstanding engineers. It is autonomous in its administration and in the selection of its members, sharing with the National Academy of Sciences the responsibility for advising the federal government. The National Academy of Engineering also sponsors engineering programs aimed at meeting national needs, encourages education and research, and recognizes the superior achievements of engineers. Dr. Wm. A. Wulf is president of the National Academy of Engineering.

The **Institute of Medicine** was established in 1970 by the National Academy of Sciences to secure the services of eminent members of appropriate professions in the examination of policy matters pertaining to the health of the public. The Institute acts under the responsibility given to the National Academy of Sciences by its congressional charter to be an adviser to the federal government and, upon its own initiative, to identify issues of medical care, research, and education. Dr. Harvey V. Fineberg is president of the Institute of Medicine.

The **National Research Council** was organized by the National Academy of Sciences in 1916 to associate the broad community of science and technology with the Academy's purposes of furthering knowledge and advising the federal government. Functioning in accordance with general policies determined by the Academy, the Council has become the principal operating agency of both the National Academy of Sciences and the National Academy of Engineering in providing services to the government, the public, and the scientific and engineering communities. The Council is administered jointly by both Academies and the Institute of Medicine. Dr. Bruce M. Alberts and Dr. Wm. A. Wulf are chair and vice chair, respectively, of the National Research Council.

www.national-academies.org

Preface and Acknowledgments

I n 1997, as the 15-year term of the Lucille P. Markey Charitable Trust neared its end, the Trust approached the National Academies to conduct an evaluation of its major programs in biomedical science. The Academies agreed to undertake a project evaluating Markey Trust programs that supported the education and research of predoctoral students in clinical research, promising young biomedical investigators in postdoctoral and junior faculty positions, and senior researchers in the basic biomedical sciences. For a more complete description of the Markey Trust and some of its activities, please refer to *Bridging the Bed-Bench Gap: Contributions of the Markey Trust*, published by the National Academies Press in 2004.

The Markey Trust supported postdoctoral fellows, especially at their time of transition to junior faculty, through two programs:

• *Scholar Awards in Biomedical Sciences*. By establishing the Markey Scholars program in 1984, the Trustees recognized that top priority should be given to the support of young researchers as they moved from postdoctoral into junior faculty positions. The goal was to enable the Scholars to conduct independent research early in their careers. Between 1985 and 1991, a total of 113 Markey Scholars were supported for up to 3 years of postdoctoral training followed by 5 years as beginning faculty members. This support included both salary and research funding.

- *United Kingdom and Australian Visiting Fellows.* In addition to the Scholars program, the Trustees supported outstanding young scientists from the United Kingdom and Australia by enabling them to spend 2 years as postdoctoral fellows at American research institutions. A total of 36 Visiting Fellows—26 from the United Kingdom and 10 from Australia—were selected between 1986 through 1994.

This is the second of five reports to emerge from the evaluation of the Markey Trust. As part of its assessment of the Markey Trust, the NRC hosted a scientific conference for Markey Scholars and Visiting Fellows in Rio Grande, Puerto Rico on June 28-30, 2002. The purpose of the conference was to enable the Scholars and Fellows to share their research experiences, just as they did at the annual Scholars Conferences previously conducted by the Markey Trust. All of the attending Scholars and Fellows submitted abstracts of their poster sessions. Six scholars, along with other experts in the biomedical sciences, made formal presentations. The report contains two sections and a set of appendixes. The first section presents selected formal papers presented at the conference both by invited guests and by selected Markey Scholars. The second section presents abstracts of the scientific poster sessions. The appendixes present conference-related material on the agenda and participants. The statements made in the enclosed papers are those of the individual authors and do not necessarily represent positions of the National Research Council (NRC).

This volume has been reviewed in draft form by individuals chosen for their technical expertise, in accordance with procedures approved by the NRC's Report Review Committee. The purpose of this independent review is to provide candid and critical comments that will assist the institution in making its published report as sound as possible and to ensure that the report meets institutional standards for quality. The review comments and draft manuscript remain confidential to protect the integrity of the process.

We wish to thank the following individuals for their review of the selected papers: Wendy Baldwin, University of Kentucky; Wendy Havran, The Scripps Research Institute; David Hockenbery, Fred Hutchinson Cancer Research Institute; Agnes Kane, Brown University; and Peter Scacheri, National Institutes of Health.

Although the reviewers listed above have provided constructive comments and suggestions, they were not asked to endorse the content of the individual papers. Responsibility for the final content of the papers rests with the individual authors.

The project was aided by the invaluable help of the BHEW professional staff—George R. Reinhart, senior project officer; Elaine Lawson, project officer; Stacey Kozlouski, research assistant, Elizabeth Briggs Huthnance, administrative assistant, and Heather Begg, program assistant.

Enriqueta Bond, Chair
Committee on the Evaluation of the Lucille P. Markey
Charitable Trust Programs in Biomedical Sciences

Contents

Selected Invited
Conference Papers

Update on Markey Scholars

Krystyna Isaacs, Ph.D.
SciConsult

The Markey Trust funded seven classes of scholars. This paper presents a description of the first five classes of Markey Scholars, those who received their initial funding between 1985 and 1989.

Over three-fourths of the scholars from classes 1 to 5 are employed at academic institutions, 12 percent are at non-profit research facilities such as Scripps, 8 percent are at for-profit research facilities such as Merck, and 3 percent are in professions not directly involved in research or medicine.

Of those in academia, roughly one-third are now full professors, two-thirds are associate professors, and one is a senior member. And of those in the private or non-profit sector, 13 hold positions such as president, or director, or senior member.

We calculated publication rates as the total number of articles published over the entire life of the scholar. Productivity ranged from a low of 10 to a high of 180, with an average of 53 peer-reviewed articles published.

The National Research Council generates ranking tables on science departments at public and private academic institutions. They have identified the top-ten institutions in the fields of cellular and developmental biology, biochemistry and molecular biology, and molecular and general genetics. These top-ranked programs are in a total of 13 universities. Nearly 60 percent of the scholars in academia are employed at one of those 13 universities.

As part of the overall evaluation of the Markey Scholars conducted by the National Research Council, we are conducting ethnographic interviews with all scholars. While this part of the evaluation is not analytic, it provides useful information on the scholars. Interviews are scheduled approximately 10–12 years following the receipt of the Markey award and consist of 30 to 45 minute telephone conversations. A thorough and complete evaluation of the Markey Scholars program will be published by National Academies Press in the summer of 2005 and can be viewed on the National Academies web site: www.nationalacademies.org.

The interviews began with several general topics. Questions were raised regarding how and why decisions were made. The first question was, "Remember, way back when you were a lowly fellow or a postdoc. How did you even find out about the award, and how did you feel when you got the phone call from Bob Glaser?" Many of the scholars said they heard about this award through their mentor, the department chair, or their advisor. This is especially true for the first two or three classes, when the Markey Trust was a new program and had not received much publicity. Later the "postdoc/fellows grapevine" started to play a larger role in publicizing the Markey Award and people responded to posted notices.

One of the first questions we asked was whether the additional postdoc year requirement was onerous. Some of the scholars believed they were ready to leave when they got the award, but others felt the additional year gave them time to wrap up experiments, collect sufficient data for those reports and grants they needed to write, and also to do job interviews.

A number of scholars mentioned that the award gave dual-career scientific couples time to get their career stages in sync. Many scholars were married or were about to be married to other scientists or other medical professionals, and they were either 1 to 2 years behind or 1 to 2 years ahead of their spouse. This extra time helped to get these dual-career couples on the same path, and it also aided in job hunting.

Many scholars mentioned that the Markey award gave them confidence to pursue riskier lines of investigation. Not that they changed the direction of their research program or changed their ideas, but these scholars felt like they had the ability to pursue research that would never be funded by the NIH without significant amounts of pilot data.

Many scholars learned about jobs through the annual scholars conferences. As scholars wandered through the hall, networking and talking with other scholars, conference speakers, reviewers, or other people invited to the conference, they frequently were informed of potential job openings.

We were also curious to learn what variables influenced the choices of those who changed locations vs. those who did not. Follow-up questions indicated that for many scholars, spouses' job requirement played an important role in relocation plans. Scholars volunteered that this was critical to them; they were married to a professional and they were not about to drag him/her off into a situation where the spouse could not work. They used the time and the flexibility that the scholar award gave them to find the perfect job for both. Other important considerations were the quality of the graduate student population, the scholar's particular research interest, reputation of the department, and the economics of the geographical region.

A number of scholars spoke up about their startup package and the negotiation experience. Those who stayed at their fellowship institution had significantly less funds in their startup packages. This was not surprising. The scholar was already in-place, so the institutions saw no need to offer them a substantial start-up package.

Once scholars assumed faculty status, we wanted to know about their life as junior faculty—what kind of pressures they had from the department to do something other than research, so-called "departmental expectations." We found that in general scholars had very light committee loads. Many scholars mentioned they wanted to be active members in the department, so some actually volunteered for more committee work than was required.

Teaching was never a focus of the Markey Scholars Award; there were no teaching requirements attached to the fellowship. As scholars climbed the career ladder they assumed more administrative duties and many took on more teaching responsibilities than they originally had. Generally speaking, M.D.s and M.D.-Ph.D.s at medical institutions have very light teaching loads compared to colleagues with Ph.D.s at basic research institutions. Markey Scholars are no different.

It is a sign of the times that a significant number of scholars have a commercial interest in science. We found many scholars had patents, collaborated with industry, sat on the board of directors or the scientific advisory board for a biotech company, and/or had started their own biotech company.

Over and over again the scholars repeated that what they loved was the fact that the Markey Trust had faith in them as a person, not as a project, but in *them*. They really appreciated the lack of bureaucracy and the fact that administrative decisions were made on a timely basis. Many of the scholars believed that the success of the Markey Scholars program was based on the length of the funding. Seven years of guaranteed funding offered the scholars job security, and the scholars really understood how much this helped them and enabled them to engage in risky science. The scholars also thought the annual conferences were important. Some scholars that left to go to industry, biotech, or Howard Hughes Medical Institute (HHMI) felt shut out that they were not invited to subsequent conferences. Finally, scholars were asked, "What could you do to make the program stronger or better? After a long pause, most responded that the program should not have ended after only seven cycles.

Two quotes from the scholars best summarize how they felt about the Markey Trust.

The first one is:

> One of most important aspects was not the dollars, but a feeling of protection in some way and camaraderie both between the participants and the people who were involved in the trust. What I'd like to convey is not just the idea that it was great to give people lots of dollars, but that it was equally important to address the welfare of the scholars. Money alone is not what it is about.

And the second one is:

> I have warm feelings about the Trust. The only thing on my office wall is my Markey certificate.

Ensuring the Future Participation of Women in Science, Mathematics, and Engineering

Shirley M. Tilghman, Ph.D.
Princeton University

The title of this paper is *"Ensuring the Future Participation of Women in Science, Mathematics, and Engineering"* because those are the three main areas that I want to address. Over the past 25 years, there has been remarkable progress in the participation of women in all of these fields. We should celebrate that fact, and not let it get lost.

Why is it important that women are active participants in science, engineering, and mathematics? There are four arguments that suggest why we should care. The first argument is that science will benefit the scientific community by tapping into the entire talent pool. If we are only encouraging half of the population to enter careers in science, we are losing an enormous potential. The second argument, which is debatable, is that women's interests in science may not completely coincide with the kinds of things that interest men. Women do not do science differently; rather, their interests may differ in some cases. By encouraging women to enter into science, we increase the diversity of the kinds of problems that we study in science. The third argument is unquestionably true. Science will look increasingly anachronistic if women do not participate. As women's participation increases in every other activity, science will be less attractive in general to talented students without active participation by women. Finally, it is unjust for a profession to organize itself in such a way as to exclude women; it is a pure justice argument.

If we examine the 25-year period from 1975 to 2001, there has been a steady increase in the number of women completing bachelor's degrees in all branches of science. In biological sciences and in chemistry women are essentially at parity. Fifty percent of the bachelor's degrees in those fields currently are being awarded to women. In the physical sciences women's participation is lagging, but has more than doubled in the 25-year period. Nineteen percent of bachelor's degrees in physics are awarded to women as are 18 percent of undergraduate engineering degrees.

There has been a steady increase in the number of women completing Ph.D.s in all of the sciences. In biological sciences, women now earn over 40 percent of doctorates, and in chemistry a remarkable 33 percent of doctorates are awarded to women; that is a three-fold increase in 25 years. In the physical sciences, 12 percent of doctoral degrees are awarded to women and in engineering there has been a five-fold increase, from an unbelievable 2 percent in 1975 up to 11 percent in 2001.

In addition, women are entering the faculty in increasing numbers. The number of women in science faculty has been increasing at every rank. However, one of the chronic problems in women's distribution across ranks in academia is that women are most dominant in the instructor/lecturer position. At most institutions these tend to be non-tenure track positions with the least job security. Some of the differences between assistant, associate, and full professors can be explained by pipeline issues. Although the pipeline is increasingly becoming a problematic excuse for the small number of women in the full professor ranks and cannot be used as excuse anymore. There is clearly leakage as one moves up the professional ranks to full professor.

One could celebrate these numbers. One could say that these numbers are telling us that it is simply a matter of time. That if we gather together in another 10 years, we will see further progress and eventually women will be full and equal participants in science, engineering, and mathematics. That we are on a good track; let us just keep going. That there need not be any additional attention paid to this issue; this is a time-dependent phenomenon.

This argument cannot be supported. In fact, there are a number of indicators that suggest that unless we continue to focus on this issue we are at risk not of just stalling out, but of actually falling back. Here are some of the indicators that give me pause.

In 1999, women full professors were concentrated in non-research intensive academic institutions. In 2-year institutions (these are community and junior colleges), 42 percent of full professors were women. In liberal arts colleges (these are colleges without a graduate school), 23 percent of full professors were women. In the research-intensive university, 17 percent of full professors were women. Women Ph.D.s are not distributed evenly across different kinds of academic institutions; rather, they are in the places where one is least likely to find women at the top of the professoriate.

Thirty-four percent of women scientists and engineers are unmarried compared to 17 percent of men. Ten percent of married women scientists and engineers have an unemployed spouse compared to 38 percent of men. Twenty-one percent of women scientists and engineers identified balancing family and work as a career obstacle compared to 2.8 percent of men. That may be the most important finding as it reflects the other two. These data state loudly and clearly that the professional experience of women in science and engineering is substantively different than it is for men in the same field. As we examine all the issues, I come back to this fundamental difference in the experience of men and women.

The study initiated at the Massachusetts Institute of Technology (MIT) several years ago by Nancy Hopkins has now been replicated at several other institutions, including Cal Tech. The reports have shown that women in science and engineering faculty are more likely to report that they feel marginalized and isolated at their institution, have less job satisfaction, have unequal lab space, unequal salary, unequal recognition through awards and prizes, unequal access to university resources, and unequal invitations to take on important administrative responsibilities, especially those that deal with the future of the department or the research unit. The fact that this study has been replicated at other institutions says that this is not an MIT specific problem. This is a generalized problem about the way women faculty at research-intensive universities experience their career environment.

All of these phenomena suggest that this is an issue that has not gone away. We cannot let the numbers run. We need to do some careful thinking about what are the underlying forces that impact these indicators.

Here are some of the forces that we have to contend with, and it is important that we state them openly and clearly, and not pretend they are not important issues.

The first and largest force is the cultural expectation that women have primary-care responsibilities. Obviously, they have the biological responsibility of bearing the child, but in fact even after the child is born women are expected by society to take on the primary responsibility of childcare. There have been many fascinating studies that have looked at the impact over the past 25 years of what is clearly a very positive movement of men wanting to be more engaged in parenthood. All of those studies say that improvements in fact are there, that men are much more engaged in childcare than they used to be. But all of those studies also say that the balance is still very unequal, that women still assume the greatest amount of responsibility. After children leave the home, women also become the primary caretaker of elderly parents.

Another force—that is important when you consider point number one—is the intensification of work expectations in all job sectors. There are many current studies that show that the workforce in America is taking fewer leisure hours. The amount of hours at work is increasing. The 40-hour workweek has been replaced by a 48-hour workweek. The average number of weeks of vacation that we take is declining across the country. So this intensification, this increasing expectation of what is required in order to do the job, is a force that is really working against the further inclusion of women into science and engineering.

The increasing length of both graduate and postgraduate training is a trend that disadvantages women enormously. It disadvantages men as well. It serves no one's interest to have Ph.D. and postdoctoral training now upwards of a dozen years before becoming an independent investigator and running their own laboratory. The coincidence of these years with childbearing makes it more difficult for women to contemplate, to anticipate that they in fact can have a successful scientific career.

This issue is especially important in the physical sciences, mathematics, and engineering where there is a paucity of good role models and mentors. Both of these forces are important. In fields where they are few women it has become a vicious circle. Generating numbers really matters. It is becoming less of an issue in the biological sciences where there are so many women doing well, but for science, physical sciences, and mathematics this is a serious issue.

Finally, there is another cultural norm that we have to fight against, which is the norm that sets no expectations for women's success in science and devalues women's contribution. There are many studies that have shown that women are given cues — beginning in high school, extending into college and graduate school, and even into postdoctoral studies—that women need not set high expectations. These cues come from important people such as mentors, professors, and colleagues that say, "Well, you don't *really* have to try and get a job in a research-intensive university. Why don't you think more about going to, you know, a small teaching college. Wouldn't you have a nicer life that way?" It is very important that we are conscious of the cues that we send to our women students because they are picking them up. Without high expectations, people very quickly become discouraged. This is a chronic problem, and one that we must be conscious of and fight against.

There is no magic bullet; one thing that would get us on a straightforward path that would need very little correction. There are, however, examples of best practices, things that we in our own institutions can do that will increase the likelihood that our students and fellows will go on to have the kind of successful careers in science that all of you in this room have enjoyed so enormously.

The first best practice is articulating the value of diversity, and then rewarding it. At Princeton this year I established a fund in the provost's office that would create supplementary positions in any department who could bring to an interdisciplinary committee or faculty, a candidate who would increase the diversity of our faculty. Princeton is no different than any of the rest of your institutions. We have fewer women than should be on the faculty. We certainly have fewer African-Americans than we should have on our faculty. We established carrots in the provost's office that reward diversity in hiring with supplementary positions for the life of the time the hire works at the university. As a consequence of this, Princeton hired four senior-level African-American scholars in different fields this year. That represents 50 percent of the total number that were in the university prior to that. Clearly articulating this as a priority and providing resources for its completion can prove very successful. As a result of this program, we are hiring two women in civil engineering, the first two in that department. We are hiring a woman in mathematics, and we are hiring a woman in physics. Stating that the goals are important and giving resources can lead to good progress.

The second best practice is obvious. Institutions have to have family-friendly policies. One of the best conversations I have had in the last 6 months was with Gerry Rubin, who spoke at Princeton last month about the new Howard Hughes Medical Institute (HHMI) initiative, Janelia Farm. The question that Gerry posed to me is, "Here we have this opportunity to create an entirely new institution, how can we create it in such a way that it will be a great place for women to work?" The fact that Gerry would ask that question had me smiling for weeks afterwards. The fact that I think he is going to succeed at it made me even happier.

There are many family-friendly policies that we all know about. We have to make sure that they are in place, and that they are being administered fairly. We cannot ignore the fact that while women faculty, women scientists, and women engineers are having small children, they are going to be less productive; during that period, they are working two jobs. The only way that institutions can compensate for this is to implement what we should be doing across the board, which is recognizing quality, not quantity. In the end, what pushes science forward? It is not the 22 papers in Biochemical and Biophysical Research Communications (BBRC). What pushes science forward are the seminal papers, the extraordinarily creative, imaginative, groundbreaking piece of work. If we as a field reward quality and not quantity, women at all stages of their careers will compete extremely effectively.

Mentoring is important and it is important at every level. Arthur Miller said, "Attention must be paid." This is important, it has been shown over and over, and over again, how important mentoring is at the undergraduate level. The institutions that do the best at encouraging women to enter careers in science are the small liberal arts colleges and the historically black colleges. Spellman College sends more black women into science than the rest of universities put together. The reason is that these are institutions that pay a lot of attention to individuals. For young women to be interested in science, what really matters is being in a place where people are paying attention to people. Of course, this extends up through the ranks as well.

Institutions have to take the lead that was set by MIT and study themselves, and then honestly publicize the results. We need to know where we are in order to know where we are going. I really admire Chuck Vest at MIT. He did an extraordinary thing by publishing the results of that MIT study. He set a model that the rest of the universities should absolutely be following.

The last point is developing curriculum that encourages students rather than weeds them out, but at the same time that also sets high expectations.

For example, this year I met with the advisory committee to our computer science department. Computer science is a very interesting field because it was created about the same time as molecular biology. One of the explanations that has been given for why there are so many women in molecular biology relative to other sciences is because it was a new field; it did not have 250 years of culture dragging along behind it. From the very outset women were active participants and it was the lack of history that really made the difference. Computer science is a counter example. Computer science started just about the same time and had a similar early history. Women poured into computer science in the 1960s, and were doing extremely well and then their numbers took a nosedive. Now computer science is a field that struggles to find women students.

The advisory committee pointed something out to me. Imagine what it is like for a woman on the first day of a Computer Science 101 class. She is sitting in a room full of young men who have been programming since they were 12, spending their entire lives in their bedrooms playing computer games, and who can probably *teach* the class. There are very few young women who come in with that kind of cultural background. There are fundamental differences in the experiences of 18-year-old men and women with respect to computer science. It is extremely important to create curriculum that is equally satisfying to men and women rather than putting them in the same classes and expecting the same outcomes from them. For about 4 years, Carnegie Mellon has had a program in place that does exactly that, and it has been extraordinarily successful. They are now graduating more women in computer science than any other university in the country. It was simply a matter of acknowledging this simple difference, and then adjusting the curriculum.

These are some of the things that we are trying to do in order to ensure that the next generation of scientists, engineers, and mathematicians is going to include women.

The Future of Non-profit Funding in Biomedical Research

Gerald M. Rubin, Ph.D.
Howard Hughes Medical Institute

This presentation is about the future of all non-profit funding for biomedical research. This is a huge topic, and beyond my ability to address. One particular institution, the Howard Hughes Medical Institute (HHMI), happens to be the largest non-profit funder of biomedical research in the United States.

Funding from non-profits is very small compared to federal funding. The Hughes' budget is about 2 to 3 percent of the total National Institutes of Health (NIH) budget, and about 5 percent of NIH funding for basic biomedical research. So even though we are the largest non-profit funder in biomedical research in the country, we are still small compared to the NIH. It is important that non-profits distinguish themselves from the NIH by being less risk-adverse. Once something becomes established, we should let the government fund it and move on. Another difference is that organizations like the HHMI and, to a large extent, the Markey Trust, unlike the NIH, tend to fund people, not projects. That is, they identify individuals who are talented, and give them money and freedom to pursue their own initiatives.

HHMI has an annual budget of $650 million. We are required by law to spend 3.5 percent of our net worth every year and we actually spend over 5 percent. In 2001, this amounted to about $515 million for medical research, $100 million for grant programs, and the remainder for administrative and other incidental costs. The grant expenditures are spread across a number of programs, including support for undergraduate science education in the United States, biomedical research in a number of foreign countries with limited resources, fellowships for graduate students and fellowships for M.D.s to get postdoctoral research training after they complete their M.D. degree. However, we are phasing out the latter program because the NIH has instituted awards that do the same thing. We are delighted to let the NIH take over this activity while we pursue other approaches to funding physician scientists. If the NIH imitates us, it is the sincerest form of flattery.

With regard to funding for medical research, 80 percent goes directly to HHMI Investigators. There are now 325 investigators at 72 institutions in the United States. The rest is controlled from HHMI headquarters in the form of space and overhead payments to the host institutions, and for major equipment items, which are given out separately to investigators.

As the endowment increased from about $5 billion back in 1986 to a little over $11 billion today, the number of investigators has increased from 96 to a planned plateau of 330, however, there have been as many as 348. Some investigators leave to assume administrative jobs, or jobs in biotech or academia, which requires them to give up their appointment. In addition, we review our own investigators every 5 years, and about 20 percent are not renewed. These two sources of attrition are about the same magnitude. We have periodic competitions where we appoint new investigators.

This was the situation two and a half years ago when Tom Cech took over as president of HHMI, and recruited David Clayton and me as vice presidents. We began to evaluate how the Institute spends its money to determine what changes would be appropriate for the future. When we started this examination the endowment had just gone through a period of rapid growth. We agreed that even if the endowment continued to grow, it would not make sense to increase the number of investigators to 400. There are two reasons for this conclusion.

The first was that we know our investigators as individuals because the bureaucracy is not large. Our organization had already been strained with 330 investigators. To increase to 400 would mean that we could not maintain our style of review, and personal interaction. Moreover, at this time, the NIH was providing generous funding for many scientists. We felt that if we increased the number of investigators to 400, the best we could hope for was a 15 percent increase in the output. That did not seem like the best way to spend money. The primary mission of HHMI is to fund and advance basic biomedical research in the United States. Our challenge was to determine the best way to use this additional money.

We anticipated additional funds of $50 million to $60 million. The cost of an investigator, if you include the money that is given to the host institution in payments for rent and utilities, is about $1.2 million per year. Not all the investigators are in this range, but that is the average.

Based on this number, $50 million to $60 million, would allow us to employ and support the work of 40-50 new investigators. Did we want to increase the number of investigators or do something else with these funds?

In addition, we saw an advantage to having some of our programs not closely tied to our 70 host institutions, although there are clearly many advantages of working with host institutions. One is that we spend money efficiently when we house our investigators at host institutions because, although they become Hughes' employees, they stay fully integrated members of the host institution, benefiting from its infrastructure. Taking advantage of the host institution's infrastructure ensures that we can maximize the amount of research conducted. This is a huge advantage. So we anticipate keeping 80 to 90 percent of our research program in this mode. On the other hand, host institutions have their own culture and HHMI investigators must be part of that culture. Consequently, there are a number of factors that HHMI cannot influence, such as tenure decisions.

These considerations led us to decide that rather than simply increase the number of investigators tied to individual host institutions we would set up a free-standing independent research center. We wanted to have a critical mass, and to have that critical mass associated with one or a small number of host institutions would upset the balance of our ongoing relationships. That said, we also wanted to avoid duplicating what we do successfully in collaboration with our host institutions. We did not want simply to create another Whitehead or Salk Institute, despite the fact that these are highly successful research institutions—and ones that each house several of our investigators. These are great places, but they function much like university departments.

We found ourselves in a very unusual situation; we had a clean slate, no rules, and sufficient money to do something, but had not figured out what would be best to do. Two decades ago the Markey Trust found itself in a similar position. We began to examine issues that are particular to the current American biomedical research enterprise.

First, there is a lack of places for scientists who want to continue to work in the lab with their own hands. Most scientists start as someone else's graduate student and they serve an apprenticeship as a postdoc in someone else's lab. As postdocs, they have varying degrees of independence, depending on the lab. They do that for several years, and then assume a faculty position and run their own lab. Especially in top-tier institutions, young faculty are increasingly advised not to work in the lab themselves, but to build a sizable research group with more hands doing more work publishing more papers. In many institutions, even medical schools with low teaching loads, the average assistant professor is out of the lab within a year or two. While this may increase productivity and be an appropriate mode of operating for the vast majority of scientists, it is not ideal for the minority who do not really fit into this mold. This was an unmet need that we thought we could address.

Second, the length of time spent in training—or worse, indentured servitude—has increased substantially in the last two decades. When I was a postdoc in the mid-1970s at Stanford, there was a big debate in the biochemistry department of whether to permit a third postdoctoral year, or if 2 years was the maximum amount of postdoc time before assuming independence. The extended postdocs of today were very rare back then. I became an assistant professor at the age of 26. The other two people hired in the same year in my department were also 26. Now people generally do not become assistant professors until they are much older, especially those with M.D.s. Even Ph.D.s are age 30 and over when they achieve independence.

These forces conspire such that there is little or no period at the top-tier institutions when scientists are both truly independent and afforded the time to be able to work in their lab with their own hands. There have also been changes in the culture of academic institutions in the award of tenure and expectations about publications that penalize small groups.

In addition, we observed that there was no place for groups of people from different institutions to come together and collaborate. It is common for an individual to do a sabbatical in someone else's lab. What is very uncommon is for three or four people to get together and collaborate in research. Imagine three people went walking on the beach and one of them said, "If there were someplace we could get together for a year, each bringing half a dozen members of our lab, and someone would give us money, we could try this crazy idea, and see if it works." There is currently no place you can do this, and nobody would fund it. This is another unmet need we thought we could address by developing an institution that would reserve a reasonable amount of space, perhaps a third, for visiting scientists who would submit proposals for interesting scientific projects and come together on the project, which we would fund.

To achieve these goals we would both include and reach outside our own set of investigators. At the same time we would provide a place to nurture creative individuals that do not fit in the current system. Many excellent scientists do not excel in the non-scientific skills needed to be successful in the typical academic setting. When you get your own lab you are required to do things for which you were not trained and have nothing to do with research. It is like running a small business. You have to hire people, fire people, evaluate individuals, motivate people, recruit graduate students, lure postdocs to your lab, and deal with their personal problems. Some people who would function extremely well as research scientists, do not excel in these other things. They have difficulty making the transitions necessary to succeed as independent investigators in typical academic settings and might do much better in an environment where they could concentrate more fully on research.

As an example, here is a self-assessment by one of these "impaired" individuals:

> "I have indeed actively tried to avoid both teaching and administrative work. This was partly because I thought I would be no good at them, but also out of selfishness. I do not enjoy them, whereas I find research most enjoyable and rewarding."

> "Of the three main activities involved in scientific research, thinking, talking and doing, I much prefer the last and am probably best at it. I am all right at thinking, but not much good at the talking."

> "'Doing' for a scientist implies doing experiments, and I managed to work in the laboratory as my main occupation from when I started as a Ph.D. student until I retired. Unlike most of my scientific colleagues, I was not academically brilliant. …However, when it came to research where experiments were of paramount importance and fairly narrow specialization was helpful, I managed to hold my own ..."

By his own assessment, this person would not have done well as an assistant professor in most institutions, but in actuality he managed to do very well. This quote is from an autobiographical essay by Fred Sanger (*Ann. Rev. Biochem.* [1988] 57:1-28), who, as many of you know, was the only person to win the Nobel Prize twice in chemistry, first for devising methods for sequencing proteins and then for sequencing DNA.

There is a need for places for people who are very creative and want to muddle about in the lab with their own hands for their entire career; such individuals do not really fit into most academic institutions. There are places, like the NIH, where scientists can do this. In this sense we are not inventing anything new. Our goal is to create a home for people who want to be directly involved in the conduct of research with a small research group of their own without the distractions of grant writing, teaching, committee work, and other administrative responsibilities. The way you build critical mass for larger projects in such an environment is by interacting with your colleagues to create larger, perhaps interdisciplinary, groups.

Let me state that, for most individuals, we expect we will be providing a way to delay non-research activities rather than totally avoid them because our view is of a place where people would spend the beginning of their independent career, when they really want to work in the lab. Later, when they transition into a more typical university lifestyle, midway through their independent career, they can assume these other responsibilities.

One of the things that we hope to provide by postponing grant writing, etc., is to enable scientists to focus on science in a less pressured and an unscheduled environment. It is very, very rare in a university environment to be able to talk spontaneously with colleagues for a couple of hours without worrying about appointments and other time obligations. Our hope is that by getting rid of these distractions we can provide that time. Most assistant professors probably spend 30, 40, or maybe as much as 50 percent of their time not on their own scientific research, but dealing with their grants, classroom teaching, worrying about hiring support staff, and worrying about other issues. Such an environment might enable scientists to succeed while spending only 50 hours a week doing their research, rather than needing an 80-hour workweek, because we eliminated 30 hours of activities that are not directly related to their research or to interacting productively with their colleagues. That is our goal.

In addition to having a place to do this, you also need to establish a culture and a scientific program. I am going to focus mainly on the culture here because I think that, by far, it is the most difficult and the most important to develop. You can always change your research program and indeed you expect the research to change over time. But once you establish a culture, once your reputation for a given style of operation has been made, it is very difficult to change.

Here is another quote. This one is from the person who I think has been the most successful in establishing a culture in a research institution. This is from Max Perutz (from the Preface to *I Wish I'd Made You Angry Earlier* [Cold Spring Harbor Press, NY, 2000]):

> "Every now and then I receive visits from earnest men and women armed with questionnaires and tape records who want to find out what made the Laboratory of Molecular Biology in Cambridge (where I work) so remarkably creative. They come from the social sciences and seek their Holy Grail in interdisciplinary organization. I feel tempted to draw their attention to 15th century Florence with a population of less than 50,000, from which emerged Leonardo Michelangelo, Raphael, Ghiberti, Brunelleschi, Alberti, and other great artists. Had my questioners investigated whether the rulers of Florence had created an interdisciplinary organization of painters, sculptors, architects, and poets to bring to life this flowering of great art? Or had they found out how the 19th century municipality of Paris had planned Impressionism, so as to produce Renoir, Cézanne, Degas, Monet, Manet, Toulouse-Lautrec, and Seurat? My questions are not as absurd as they seem, because creativity in science, as in the arts, cannot be organized. It arises spontaneously from individual talent. Well-run laboratories can foster it, but hierarchical organization, inflexible, bureaucratic rules, and mounts of futile paper-

work can kill it. Discoveries cannot be planned; they pop up, like Puck, in unexpected corners."

Max Perutz was the first director of the Medical Research Council Laboratory of Molecular Biology (MRC), arguably the most successful scientific biological research institution for 30 years from the 1950s to the 1980s, although I may be biased because I did my Ph.D. there. Perutz made it successful for a number of reasons. Let me point out two things about him. First was his desire to minimize bureaucracy; he ran an institution with 300 people and yet managed to spend most of his time working in his laboratory. Second, which is probably more important, was his remarkable ability for recruiting talent, nurturing that talent and not taking credit for that talent's work.

Most people in this room probably would not be aware that when Watson and Crick discovered the double helix, Watson was Perutz's postdoc and Crick was Perutz's graduate student. In fact, Crick was Perutz's second graduate student. His first graduate student was John Kendrew. Here is a scientist whose first two graduate students and first postdoc all won the Nobel Prize, less than 15 years after starting in his lab. I do not think that anyone is going to match that record, but it shows a major reason why the MRC was so successful.

So when we examined models for our institution, the MRC is one of the institutions we looked at and, for the non-biological sciences, the ATT's Bell Labs. These laboratories share some common attributes. They both had small group sizes. Their PIs work actively in the laboratory. They tend to be places where people spend part of, but not their entire career. So these are two of the most influential models we are using to guide us.

We are imagining a facility of about 400 persons, running the gamut from graduate student to technician to principal investigator. We expect a core of about 180 resident scientists and then about 120 support staff providing services ranging from the cleaning of glassware, to tissue culture to sophisticated machine shops. We will reserve about 100 spaces for visiting scientists who will work, fully funded, for periods of 3 weeks to 3 years, while retaining their primary appointment at their host institution.

We want to copy the successful arrangements at places such as the Carnegie Institution of Washington, the Whitehead Institute, and at University of California, San Francisco (UCSF), of having fellows enter right after graduate school with a non-renewable 5-year appointment so they can engage in an independent postdoc, perhaps supported by a technician or two. My friends at the Whitehead Institute indicate that this plan works well, but would be better with more fellows to reach a critical mass. So our goal is to accommodate up to 20 of these fellows.

Following the model of HHMI investigators based at our host institutions, we will have resident investigators who get research support including salaries for up to six additional individuals. The goal is to keep the group sizes small enough that people will interact and to also allow the group leader to be an active scientist. If you want to have an interactive environment, you have to have a small group size. I know of no institution that is truly interactive with large group sizes.

How do we get people to come to this facility? Why would young scientists want to come here as opposed to going to Harvard, Massachusetts Institute of Technology, or UCSF? We are not going to award tenure; I do not think an institution like this should have tenure because we are small and need the flexibility to change research areas with time. We will have an appointment cycle, similar to that which we use for our current investigators, which works quite well. This would include a review after 5 years with either a 2-year transitional period if they are unsuccessful in their review, or another 5-year appointment and the ability to come up for another review. HHMI investigators have the ability after they pass their first 5-year review to transfer their appointment to another institution. So in our case, we could say that passing the review is the substitute for tenure; you become an investigator with the right of transfer, and you can move to any of our 70 host institutions that will have you as a HHMI investigator.

We think many people might prefer to spend the first 8 to 10 years of their career in a place like this, without distractions, knowing that if they are successful they can move on to become a HHMI investigator in another institution. Indeed, our view is that people will not spend their whole career at the institution we will establish. We anticipate recruiting half a dozen senior scientists to provide mentorship and leadership, and those people might arrive midway in their careers and complete them here. But the idea is that most of the individuals that come here would stay for a relatively short part of their career and then move on. Although there would be the opportunity for some to stay indefinitely, they would have to embrace the small group size, the structure, and the culture of the place.

So in closing, I want to give some physical reality to this intellectual construct. We are currently in the planning phase and expect to become operational in early 2006, three and a half years from now. My primary job at HHMI is planning this new facility, and my current focus is more on the physical space and less on the culture and on the program. That is why much of what I put forth today is trial balloons and I am very open to receiving your comments.

We have purchased a piece of property, which is called Janelia Farm, and we decided to keep that name. Like Cold Spring Harbor and other similar facilities, the name will not constrain what we are doing there even into the distant future. Janelia Farm is 40 minutes by car from our headquarters. It is also 40 minutes from the White House and downtown Washington. It is only 15 minutes from Dulles Airport, which is very important for a place with a lot of visitors. We are close enough to a major metropolitan center to accommodate two-career families. Our proximity to Dulles Airport means we are within a few hours of any major, scientific center in the world. It is slightly isolated in the sense that it is not on a university campus. We view the isolation as an advantage. In my experience, interdisciplinary collaboration is counterintuitive at a place like Berkeley. It does not happen because departments are insular. While it helps to have a great computer science department on campus because my graduate students can take the programming classes necessary to do bioinformatics, in my experience the computer scientists are not really interested in our problems. Computer scientists have their own career structure, and the reward structure in universities penalizes interdisciplinary research. The underlying message is that if you want tenure, work in your own discipline; don't get involved in anyone else's discipline because you will lose your champions.

Figure 1 shows an aerial photograph of Janelia Farm. Its borders are Route 7 and the Potomac River. There are some existing office buildings and other buildings such as the old farmhouse. We will not utilize these buildings initially. Rather, there are plans for a building that will have about 200,000 square feet for research. We're going to have a 250-seat auditorium, a 100-seat auditorium, a conference facility, about 100 hotel rooms, and, 24 studio and 36 two-bedroom apartments on site. One way to overcome the isolation is to have external scientists come in for conferences, a strategy successfully employed by Cold Spring Harbor Laboratories.

The architect is Rafael Viñoly, who is involved with a number of science buildings. For example, he is working on the genomics building at Princeton. He has also designed the Kimmel Center for Performing Arts in Philadelphia, the David L. Lawrence Convention Center in Pittsburgh, and a number of other similar buildings.

Figure 2 shows one of the architect's conceptual drawings of the main science building. It will be built into the side of the hill, utilizing a natural slope down toward the river. The bottom floor will house most of the non-research space. The top two floors will house the labs, support and office space. Because we have 260 acres, we do not have a site problem. You could not build a building like this on most university campuses, where there is not a lot of land available, and where you may need to build an eight-story tower to fit the required square footage onto your building lot. To put things in scale, the National Institutes of Health cam-

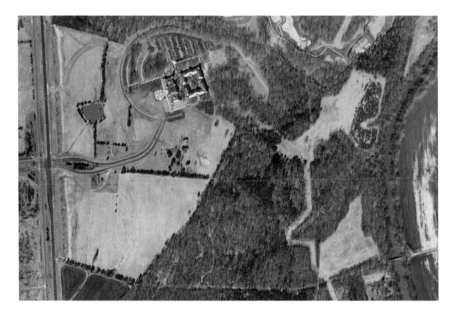

FIGURE 1 Aerial photograph of Janelia Farm.

pus is 330 acres. So we have a lot of land on which to construct a small number of buildings.

We anticipate that the program will enable people to make techno-logical advances and have access to the support staff required to develop novel instruments—a resource most academics do not have. While a num-ber of universities are developing interdisciplinary programs, there are still many problems. Until recently, the development of bioinformatics in academia was crippled because the computer scientists did not consider bioinformatics to be real computer science and the biologists did not think bioinformatics was real biology. So there was no common ground for interdisciplinary work to develop, given that individuals needed a home in either a computer science or biology department. The same thing is now happening with instrument designers and instrument builders. They do not really have a home, and one of the things we can do is create a home for them. I think that would be an important contribution.

The institution we are planning might be described by some as tech-nology focused. I do not think that is really right. I think it is an institution that is focused on unsolved problems in biology, which of necessity makes it technology driven. Unfortunately, the structure of universities limits

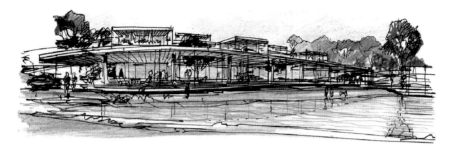

FIGURE 2 Architect's conceptual drawing of the proposed main science building.

the ability to do technology development at the required level, which may be why a lot of the most interesting technological development is happening in the private sector. I think it would be good for some of this work to return to the public sector. We hope to facilitate this by providing the kind of funding, team work, and technical support that you find now in good biotech companies, but not in the universities.

New Directions in Genomic Research

Janet D. Rowley, M.D.
University of Chicago Medical Center

Serving on the Scholar Selection Committee and the excitement of being part of an experiment in the challenging new concept for funding biomedical research was a major thrill. The Selection Committee had heated discussions about the selection criteria and whether it should follow the guidelines of half of the awards going to M.D.s and half going to Ph.D.s, or whether it should try some other combination.

The guiding hand of Purnell Choppin was critical, even though his name has not been mentioned here. He was the Chair of the Selection Committee when it first began, assisted initially by Philip Leder and then David Kipnis. It was the wisdom of Purnell that kept things on track. The Markey Scholars program has been very successful, which is a tribute to the strength of the initial guidelines, to the wisdom of the Selection Committee, and the initiative of the scholars themselves.

There are some very fundamental questions emerging from genome projects. For example, Eric Green's poster highlighted the kinds of answers that can be obtained now and from comparative genomics in the future. I am going to focus on a particular question related to genome research; one that is being raised now by comparing RNA transcripts that we can detect experimentally and that we can map to genomic DNA that are not seen in the EST database or in the UniGene clusters. I will raise the question in the context of human leukemia because that is the area in which I have done my research. The history of the study of chromosome translocations in cancer began in 1960 with the work of Peter Nowell and David Hungerford for identifying the Philadelphia Chromosome in

Chronic Myelogenous Leukemia (CML). This was followed by the discovery in 1972 that the Philadelphia Chromosome was really a translocation of chromosomes 9 and 22. In 1984 the 9;22 translocation was cloned by Nora Heistercamp and John Grafin who identified the *Abelson (ABL)* gene on chromosome 9 and the *BCR* gene on chromosome 22. Subsequent research showed that it was a fusion gene. The final advance, in 1998, was the use of Gleevec, which has turned out to be a miraculous drug for the treatment of many patients with CML. Although the chromosome abnormality was discovered in 1960, the discovery of specific treatment did not occur until 1998, almost a 40-year gap.

We examined leukemic cells from patients with acute myelogenous leukemia, each with a specific chromosome abnormality, namely different translocations, each with a unique morphology. My assumption has always been that this unique morphology is in fact associated with unique patterns of gene expression, and the challenge has been to try to figure out what these patterns are. All the breakpoints have been cloned. At the present time, except for the 15;17 translocation, we do not have genotypic specific therapy for any of these extremely common translocations.

The challenge is how to develop the optimal treatment. This is important from the clinical standpoint because the different chromosome abnormalities have different survivals, so they have prognostic implications. A 1998 study of the Medical Research Council Laboratory of Molecular Biology (MRC) that appeared in *Blood*, showed that the survival of patients with the recurring translocations I illustrated previously is 60 to 70 percent at 5 years. Surviving patients in general tend to be younger. In contrast, patients with a complex karyotype, loss of 5 or 7, or translocations of chromosome 11 have a dismal survival. These are genotypically different types of leukemia that need different types of therapy.

This raises two issues, one of which is improved diagnosis and the other, improved treatment. It is important to inform the physician of the patient's likely prognosis, as this will influence treatment. However, we are not going to get to genotype specific treatment until we have better information about the biology of these different leukemias.

To address this issue, Jim Downing's laboratory at St. Jude has used microarray analyses in childhood acute lymphoblastic leukemia. There is a unique pattern of gene expression in each one of these chromosomely unique types of leukemia. Thus, even using only known genes we can begin to develop diagnostic chips. I emphasize that these are known genes because that is all that are on the present Affymetrix microarrays.

We have taken a different approach and we are using Serial Analysis of Gene Expression (SAGE), which was developed by Ken Kinzler, and his colleague Bert Vogelstein at Johns Hopkins Medical Center. We used 3' mRNA and translated it into cDNA. SAGE uses the NLA III enzyme, which identifies a four-base pair restriction site of CATG, and then cuts at that site, as well as at a ten-base pair sequence downstream. SAGE tags are ligated together; thus in a 500-base pair sequence you can sequence many, many SAGE tags. You can then compare the SAGE tag with the present expression map to see what your transcript really represents.

We have begun our analyses in normal hematopoietic cells. We have studied CD34+ cells, and CD15+ cells from normal bone marrow; we identified 42,000 and almost 39,000 unique SAGE tags, respectively, from more than 100,000 individual SAGE tags. Note that 44 or 45 percent are novel tags, that is, they do not match to sequences in any of the expression databases. Upon careful analysis, we have found that three quarters of the SAGE tags are present only once. Examining the distribution of novel tags, we found that there were a few unknown or novel tags in the CD34+ library, and none in the CD15+ library for very frequent SAGE tags. For the single copy tags, slightly more than 50 percent are novel tags.

We analyzed CD15+ cells in the bone marrow of leukemia patients obtained prior to treatment. We found SAGE tags in the leukemia cells that were never found in normal bone marrow. Out of just this subset of 10 SAGE tags, only two were known genes. One is matched to multiple genes, and all the rest are novel sequences. As a consequence none of these would be present on any microarray.

We plan to analyze samples from five patients with each transloca-tion to identify genes that are uniquely different and uniquely over or under expressed in a particular type of chromosome abnormality to use them as a fingerprint for diagnosis. When we have identified the unique set of SAGE sequences, we will then use this as a microarray diagnostic chip. We hope that developing a prototype of a diagnostic chip will be helpful to physicians. At the same time we will try to understand the role of these transcripts in leukemia. We hope to use this information to de-velop new therapies.

All of our SAGE tags are identified using the 3'RNA transcribed into cDNA. We can now use RT-PCR to amplify from the SAGE tags to the 3' of the gene using a SAGE tag as the specific primer and a universal primer at the 3' end, resulting in sequences several hundred base pairs in length. Using 3' sequence information, we can obtain full-length cDNA. We have analyzed 23 cDNAs at present.

In one example, we extended a novel SAGE tag, to full-length cDNA and found that it matched to chromosome 19 band q13. The predicted intron/exon boundaries are based on blast search; none of the various strategies for identifying expressed sequences in the genome such as En-semble or Genescan identified any expressed sequences.

We have been able to compare alternatively spliced genes in the two normal libraries. In a series of four genes different numbers of SAGE tags representing alternatively spliced genes were identified in CD34+ and CD15+ cells. In some cases only one form is expressed in CD15+ cells and is not expressed in CD34+ cells. In another example, the same forms are expressed, but at different levels.

It has been an uphill battle trying to persuade people that these novel tags are biologically important. We were reassured from the recent paper in *Science* from Karpanov in collaboration with Bob Strasburg at NCI, describing large-scale transcriptional activity in chromosomes 21 and 22. One of the figures in the paper illustrated the use of the chip that was developed for the DiGeorge critical region on chromosome 22. RNA was obtained from a number of different cell lines, and then hybridized to this chip, which has a complete genomic sequence for this particular region. There was substantial hybridization of the RNA from these cell lines to the genomic DNA. But there was only a single exon predicted in this area. The conclusion from the paper in *Science* was that there is possibly an order of magnitude greater number of sites of transcription, of mature cytoplasmic poly A+ RNA than can be accounted for by the current annotation of the sequence of the human genome. Our data supports the idea that about half of the SAGE tags have no match.

There are a number of possibilities as to why this occurs. Clearly, the transcripts may be derived from splicing variants of known genes. I have already shown you using our own data that we know that this is true. The transcripts are present at very low levels. We have emphasized this from our own data, but that was a point that was made in the *Science* paper. The level of RT-PCR and nested RT-PCR that they had to use to get some of these transcripts indicates that they are present at low levels. The present method of getting ESTs really mitigates against finding low level RNA copies; this suggests that we need to change some of our strategies.

Are these transcripts non-coding RNA? There has been a great deal of interest now in RNA regulating the transcription of other genes. So maybe these transcripts are present in the cell and maybe they are much more abundant than any of us might imagine, but they are there to regulate other RNA or other cellular processes that we are not aware of at the present time. However, I do think that some of the transcripts may be novel genes that are not identified using current algorithms. So the broader message, and this is just an illustration, is that there is a great deal more that we are going to learn by the comparison, not only amongst genomes, but amongst these transcribed sequences. We need to try to understand what, if any, function they have in the cell. My own interest is how they are related to the development of leukemia in these particular patients.

I want to acknowledge the people in the laboratory who have been responsible for this aspect of the research. San Ming Wang is the leader of the group. Jinjun Chen is a very clever colleague who developed the GLGI. Sangzyu Lee and Guolin Zhang are doing the leukemia libraries. Markus Muschen was a visitor from Germany, his interest is in B-cells and so he is doing SAGE on B-cells. We are also indebted to Terry Clark who undertook the challenge to transform the enormous SAGE database into something intelligible.

Papers Presented by
Markey Scholars

Functional Genomics

George D. Yancopoulos, M.D., Ph.D.
Regeneron Pharmaceuticals, Inc.

L et me begin by telling you the story about not only getting my Markey award but also why I believe I was the first recipient actually to give it back. I have to give you a little background for this. My parents were Greek immigrants whose lives were interrupted by World War II and the subsequent civil war against communism in Greece. They never got a chance to finish school and were forced to leave Greece. Like many other immigrants, they worked very hard to give their kids a better chance than they had. Toward this end they stressed education. To them education was a means to an end, and that end was a high-paying job as a doctor, lawyer, or something similar.

Needless to say, when they saw that their only son—to whom they had stressed all this education—was not achieving this end, and, in fact, had decided to become a scientist and slave away in a lab for 24 hours a day and make only $10 thousand a year, they were really disappointed.

When I received the Markey award, I thought that I might finally be vindicated, at least in my Dad's eyes. I went home to tell him about this great award, and the first thing he asked me was, "Well, how much money are you going to make?" I tried to explain to him about how hard it was to fund a lab. I explained how over the course of the 7 years, the funds would add up to lots of money for my lab and so forth and so on. He cut me right off, and he said, "*Well, but exactly how much money are **you** going to make*?" When I told him that my income was going to be about $30 thousand a year, he basically started choking up. And then when he recovered, he said that without any education whatsoever he would still be making more than his son who had been going to school for more than 25 years and had both an M.D. and a Ph.D. degree.

I tried to argue that what I was doing could end up being up really important. It might even lead to new cures for important diseases. Then he said something which I've never forgotten. He said, *"Well, if what you are doing is really so important, then maybe you should think about the fact you are in the greatest country in the world … and there are some incredible opportunities here. If what you are doing is so important, then people will pay for it."*

I have been in biotech with my partner of about 13 or 14 years now, Leonard Schleifer. The Markey contribution does not end with the award. It turns out that three of the founding board members of this company— one of them, Eric Shooter, is here—were actually on the Selection Committee for the Markey Trust. And so they were three of the strongest advocates for me leaving academia and getting involved in what was then this fly-by-night operation.

I have been at Regeneron for over 13 years, and hopefully I can convince you that things have not worked out so badly. Our initial focus at Regeneron was to identify master regulatory genes involving biological processes with potential therapeutic value, such as neurotrophic growth factors, cytokines, peptide hormones, and their receptors. From the beginning what we were doing is what is now called *"functional genomics."* We also do subtractive hybridization, or what is now called *"differential display and microarrays."*

We realized from the beginning that these sorts of platforms produced a lot of candidates. The hardest thing to do once you have these candidates identified is to understand what they are doing *in vivo*. There is really no algorithm or chip that can do that for you. It requires a lot of custom work and sophisticated biologists. From the very beginning we believed in genetic approaches, and one of the most powerful ways to understand what a gene did was to knock it out or do these reporter knock-ins where you exchange the gene of interest or do transgenics.

What we do is not that much different from what a lot of people always try to do, but there is an order and science to it. A lot of it involves developing new approaches and new technologies for each step, which we all know can go wrong at any given point. This has been a primary focus at Regeneron from its early days, whether it was to pioneer or greatly simplify techniques.

I would like to spend a moment on what I think is one of the most powerful recent approaches that we have developed that has produced a lot of biology (see Figure 1). This has to do with genetic approaches, knockouts, and reporter knockins in transgenics in particular, a technology that we have been using for only a couple of years at Regeneron. We have not published the technology yet, only the fruits of the technology.

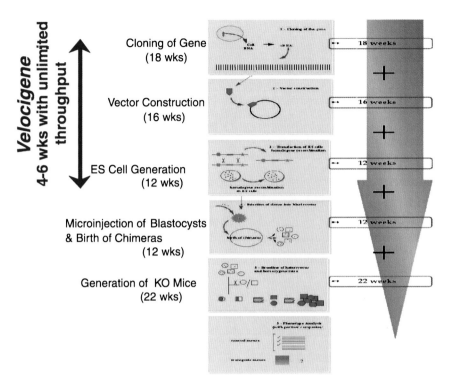

FIGURE 1 Traditional timing from a knockout service company.

This is the first truly industrialized and high precision automated way to produce knockouts and knockins in transgenics which we call "*Velocigene.*"

We make knockout constructs overnight, and within two to four weeks we have knockout mice. It's a completely automated process. What is the value of this? Well, we have hundreds, if not thousands of interesting genes we want to play with, and the thing we want to do is functionalize them. By using this Velocigene technology we can deal with things in the quantities of hundreds or thousands, which rivals what you can do in cells, worms, or fish.

The basic advantage to the bottom line is not only have we compressed the timeframe about 10-fold, but also that we can do hundreds in a period where we used to be able to do only one. I want to quickly describe some of the fruits of this technology, and show you how we can get rather dramatic, exciting data. Our goal is therapeutically interesting targets that we can eventually address to human diseases, and do translational research.

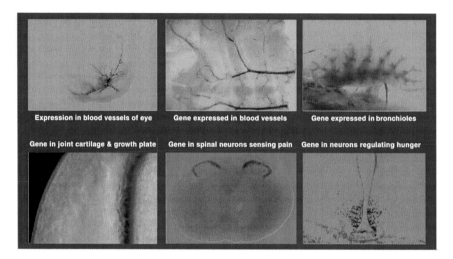

FIGURE 2 Knockouts with substitution of reporter reveal genes site of expression—unparalleled with whole body resolution, yielding clues into gene function.

We have knocked out many unknown genes or genes that have defined sequences. I want to describe some dramatic examples. We substitute reporter genes at the initiation code of the gene of interest. We have found that it almost always replicates accurately the expression pattern of the gene of interest. Our favorite method is still starting with unknown genes. We look for one that has interesting expression patterns. In Figure 2 one gene is only expressed in the blood vessels of the eye. Another gene is expressed more generally in the blood vessels. A third is expressed only in the cartilage and the growth plate or on the surface of the bone. A fourth gene has an incredibly restricted expression pattern in a single layer of neurons in the dorsal part of the spinal cord. These are neurons that sense pain, a perfect place you might want for a pain target.

We produce hundreds of these patterns, and look for the most interesting. Here in Figure 3 is a gene that is only expressed in the nerves of the teeth. Another gene is expressed in association with hair follicles and particularly with the little muscle that makes your hair stand on end. This gene is expressed widely in muscle. Another gene is in the fat that coats the mesenteric vessels, so it is a gene expressed specifically in fat. Both of these Peyer's patches are in the intestine. These are immunological structures, similar to a lymph node. And one of these genes is expressed on the outside, on the periphery of the little circular node-type structures that

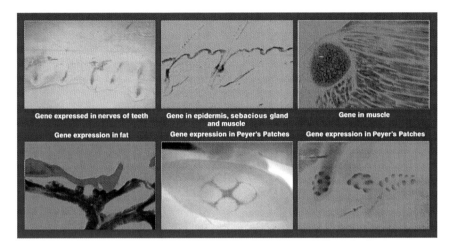

FIGURE 3 Additional gene expressions that yield clues into gene function.

you have in a Peyer's patch. This other gene is expressed actually within the central part itself, so here we have two secreted proteins that have reciprocal patterns within the same structure.

We have many genes that we have discovered that are expressed specifically in cartilage. Of the genes that are expressed in the pancreas, we have many specifically expressed secreted proteins in the pancreas. The power of this technology is that we can simultaneously be screening hundreds, if not thousands, of genes and looking for the ones that fit into specified types of patterns.

This technology is amenable to grouping genes within their site of expression, and indicating why they might be interesting and important. The data can provide important clues, and also it is incredibly pretty and dramatic as well.

We have started to put genes into classes. If we have 5 or 10 secreted proteins or their receptors that are all expressed in cartilage, we can determine if they are only expressed in cartilage or if they are actually critical master regulators of the process in which they are seemingly expressing their specificity. Not only do we do reporter knockins, but those reporter knockins we can, in a few simple steps, turn into either knockouts or into transgenics. For example, we have a growth factor receptor gene. Not only is it expressed in cartilage, but obviously it must be a critical master regulator of cartilage growth because when you knock it out, the mouse is totally devoid of cartilage. So in this manner, you define not only genes that are specific to the process that you want, but obviously the critical regulators of the process.

And why is something like this important? These are the exact cell types that degenerate, have problems, get worn out and that are not re-placed in disease of cartilage, such as in osteoarthritis. We are looking for clinically relevant targets.

We can determine that a gene, whose discovery and function was revealed by the genetic approaches in mice that I just described to you, is linked to a human disease. It turns out that in this case we were able to identify the mutation in the growth factor system that lead to cartilage growth defects in tragically involved patients. So I think it is very nice to link the gene to a patient problem, and hopefully ultimately to approaches that could help the patients.

OVER-EXPRESSION

I have shown you many genes that are expressed in blood vessels. I will now describe the discovery of a family of angiogenic factors, not only necessary but also absolutely critical for normal blood vessel formation. Instead of getting normal blood vessels patterning, when you knockout these genes you get this rather nondescript homogenous pattern.

You read about a lot of angiogenic regulators that are supposed pro-angiogenic and anti-angiogenic factors. It turns out that, in terms of ge-netic confirmation, only the Vascular Endothelial Growth Factor (VEGF) family and the family of factors known as the angiopiotiens has been genetically validated as true master regulators of blood vessel formation. Not only can we knockout these genes, but our technology is amenable to over-expressing them as well. When you over-express the same gene that in a knockout disrupts normal blood vessels, you actually get red mice. The reason the mice are red is that they have much higher densities of blood vessels. So clearly these approaches show you not only genes that are expressed in important biological processes, but that you can mediate them and that hopefully once again, these studies will have important therapeutic implications. There are a lot of diseases where the patient suffers from ischemia, low densities of blood vessels, or other settings where you want to stop blood vessel growth. I should point out this is the first genetically altered mouse by use of a growth factor that leads to stable and apparently functional and benign hyper-vascularization.

LYMPHATIC VESSEL FORMATION

Other members of this very same family that I have shown you are not necessarily involved in the same processes—they are not expressed by blood vessels. They are expressed by a different kind of vessel, lymphatic vessels. Lymphatic vessels coat the intestine, and the lacteals that dive into the villi of the intestine absorb the lipids and fats that you consume in your diet.

This gene has a very interesting expression pattern, and not only does it have an interesting expression pattern, but the knockout of this gene then ends up revealing that it is a master regulator of the process in which, once again, it is specifically expressing. So it is not a regulator of blood vessel growth, but of lymphatic vessel growth. And how do we know it? The belly of the knockout is totally filled with a milky fluid known as chyle. The knockout mouse develops huge ascites and lymphedema because it cannot absorb milk and lipids from its diet.

And why is that? This growth factor is required for the normal growth of the lymphatic vessel that allows you to absorb fat from the diet. Total disruption of the pattern, particularly of these central lacteal and lymphatics, results in a lack of absorption of this milky fluid.

Once again, genetics allows one to identify and to discover a therapeutically interesting target because if a knockout can disrupt lymphatic vessel growth, perhaps we can harness the gene to grow lymphatics in settings just like these that develop in patients where you get lymphedema.

MUSCLE FORMATION

Another biologically and therapeutically interesting area that we are interested in is muscle atrophy. We identify a lot of genes by other approaches that we thought might be specific to atrophying muscle, particularly things known as *ubiquitin ligases* that we thought could be involved in the atrophy process, because these are components of systems that degrades protein. And we thought, *"Hey, these would be perfect candidates as mediators of muscle atrophy and decay since their job is to cause degradation of protein."* The first thing that this Velocigene approach allows you to do is validate these other techniques, which are purported to identify specific genes that are activated in atrophying muscles.

The reporter knockins confirm the specificity of the muscle and their induction during atrophy. But the most important point, of course, is once again the function.

On the far left panel of Figure 4 are normal muscle fibers. In the center panel is an example of the muscle fiber size after you have induced an atrophy process such as denervation. When you knockout one of two genes, individually, you can partially rescue the atrophy. But when you do double knockouts, you almost completely prevent the atrophy (far right panel). In the double knockout you completely maintain the fiber size, showing that indeed using these approaches we can validate that we

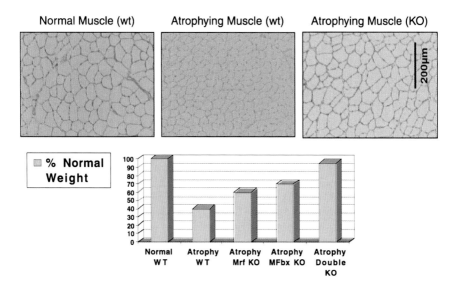

FIGURE 4 Muscle atrophy: knockouts of ubiquitin liga components proves they mediate muscle throphy.
SOURCE: Bodine et al. *Science* 294:1702; Glass et al., to be submitted.

have discovered the key-signaling components, the potential drug targets for an important process that is detrimental in a variety of human conditions.

We identified what we thought might be a key growth factor pathway that might mediate muscle growth, but how do you prove it? In this case, we did a transgenic analysis. We created a transgenic mouse that we refer to as a "mighty mouse"—all of its muscles are two to three times the normal size. We have identified genes that are involved in muscle atrophy. We knocked them out and we proved that they can prevent muscle atrophy. And we transgenically over-expressed this growth factor pathway, and we get super hypermuscularized mice.

LEAN MICE

Another example of this process is found in a transgenic of an orphan glycoprotein hormone. The epidermal fat pads in these transgenics are much smaller than normal animals. It turns out that these mice are lean. They are of normal weight, but much less of their total body weight is contributed to by fat. The thing that really is the killer for all of us is that we are exposed to a modern-day diet, which is defined as a high-fat diet. A huge percentage of the human population, and also the mouse population will get fat when fed a high-fat diet. It turns out that these lean mice, which are constituently lean on normal chow or on normal food, actually are resistant to gaining weight on high-fat diets. So on high-fat diets, control animals can gain up to 50 percent more weight. These transgenic animals essentially gained no more weight on a high-fat diet.

G-PROTEIN COUPLED RECEPTOR

This next story shows the power of the technology and how we could never even imagine going after a therapeutic target such as this, but the power of genetics reveals them to you.

We had cloned an orphan G-protein coupled receptor (GPCR), and we could never figure out where it was expressed in the body. It turns out that when we did these reporter knockins using Velocigene we found out they were expressed only in one spot in the entire body. Before birth in mammals the testes are actually not located in the scrotum, but in the mid part of the body. There is a ligamentous-type structure called the gubernaculum that is attached to the testes. The most common congenital abnormality in males is actually failure of descent of the testes because this gubernaculum has not contracted. Now, I have to admit I did not even know what a gubernaculum was when we did this Velocigene knockout, but when we saw this expression pattern in something only expressed in one spot, what we realized was it was staining only the gubernaculum. Maybe we have discovered a gene involved in this process. That was the case because when we knocked out this gene, we got failure of descent of the testes. In knockout mice, the testes remain halfway up the body where they originally started because this GPCR is the peptide receptor that regulates gubernaculum contraction and descent of the testes. Once again, we got a totally unexpected potential therapeutic target.

We use powerful approaches and exploit them intentionally to identify and functionalize interesting gene products, and reveal therapeutic opportunities.

AXOKINE

We have taken things to the next step. The types of approaches that we have been at now for more than a decade have actually yielded some very exciting drugs that are in our pipeline. One drug known as Axokine, for obesity and diabetes, is in the final stages of testing in patients.

Many of you have heard about leptin. It turns out that Axokine works via a leptin-like receptor and signaling pathway, but it works even in so-called leptin-resistant mice. Leptin travels from the fat in the body to a key brain region known as the arcuate nucleus, and acts as a physiological regulator of body weight. When you have mice or humans that are deficient in leptin they become grotesquely obese. Giving leptin to these genetically leptin-deficient mice and humans causes dramatic weight loss. The only problem is that most obesity from which at least western man suffers from is diet-induced, not genetic in nature. All of this diet-induced obesity is leptin-resistant. So when you give leptin to animals or humans who are suffering from diet-induced obesity, it has almost no effect.

We started studying Axokine for a totally different reason. Axokine is a reengineered version of a naturally occurring neurotrophic factor known as CNTF. We started studying it as a neurotrophic factor, but found rather accidentally that it was causing weight loss when given to animals and to humans. So we did a lot more work on Axokine—including cloning its receptor and understanding the signaling pathway by which it worked.

We realized that Axokine is a distant leptin relative. It uses the receptor that is a close homologue of the leptin receptor, and this receptor is expressed in the same key brain region, the arcuate nucleus, as is the leptin receptor. Because the receptor is so similar, it activates the same exact intracellular signaling pathways—the STAT3 pathway that we initially characterized for the CNTF system. Axokine is really a leptin surrogate, but its big advantage is that it superactivates this brain region. It activates the leptin-like STAT3 response in studies of leptin resistance causing known activation, but most importantly, weight loss.

Genetics, once again, provide some of the strongest validation for this in terms of the knockouts and the transgenics of both Axokine and leptin. When you give patients or animals a protein, the arcuate nucleus is about the only part of the brain that the proteins can actually access, because almost the rest of the brain is behind a blood-brain barrier. This is where these types of proteins get in, and this is the part of the brain that seems to sample the periphery and respond to weight stimuli and so forth. Both leptin and Axokine share the ability to activate the arcuate nucleus. In the arcuate nucleus these two hormones do almost exactly the same thing in the same part of the brain.

In the leptin-resistant, diet-induced models, leptin does not do anything to this part of the brain. In the leptin-resistant study where you just give the mouse a high-fat diet, the equivalent of putting him on a McDonald's-like diet, leptin has no effect. Axokine does induce weight loss, just as we predicted based on the biochemistry that I just showed you. Once again, the most important thing to us is the translation of this to humans. Everything that we have discovered and found out about how Axokine works, and what it does on animals, is starting to be confirmed and replicated in human patients in a phase-II trial in obesity.

Obesity is rapidly becoming the biggest and most dangerous epidemic facing humankind. Obesity is becoming the leading cause of preventable death in the United States today. There is essentially no satisfactory medication for it. No way to cause long-term, profound, and permanent weight loss. During treatment, we can get continuous weight loss while you are on the drug, but more importantly when you stop taking the drug, you maintain your weight loss due to Axokine. This has not been seen with any other treatment before.

After only a 3-month treatment, at the end of a year, you are more than 15 pounds below the placebo group, and the hope is that you can continue to lose even more weight if you stay on the drug longer, and we are now in the midst of the phase-III trial.

SUMMARY

I have given you a brief summary of how we have been going about doing things, and how we think this approach has led to exciting findings that might indeed have an impact on human disease. But the most important thing that I have learned after all these years is that no matter what, you still can't make your Dad happy.

Electrophysiology of Synapses

Daniel V. Madison, Ph.D.
Stanford University School of Medicine

W e have been working over the last couple of years on electro-physiology of very small populations of synapses, and what we have gleaned about learning mechanisms from those stud-ies. By way of an introduction, I want to give you a very brief and incred-ibly oversimplified view of how we think memories are made and broken in the central nervous system.

You have a brain, and when objects appear or events appear out in the world you perceive those objects. If they are important enough to you, they can cause the formation of memory trace in your central nervous system. The mechanism, by which this memory trace is thought to be formed, again in a very oversimplified way, is that the sensory input causes a high-frequency activation of neurons in your brain, which lead to the formation of a memory trace. Conversely, if those same inputs receive a sufficient amount of low-frequency activation, that can lead to the loss of the memory trace. We believe that these are models, or at least the beginnings of a model, of how one might go about retraining a memory, storing a memory, or forgetting a memory.

The models on which the people have focused over the past 10 to 20 years are known as long-term potentiation and long-term depression. Long-term potentiation is the persistent increase in synaptic strength in cortical tissues of the central nervous system. Of particular interest is the study of the hippocampus, which is the center for memory consolidation. The strength of the synaptic connection between two hippocampal pyra-midal cells is fairly stable over a long period of time. If the input that is producing that synaptic response receives a high-frequency activation, the strength of that synapse instantly strengthens, and that strength of synaptic transmission increase is persistent. This is known as long-term potentiation, and is the most compelling model that we have for how memory traces may be stored in the central nervous system at least on a fairly short-term basis of a few hours.

Conversely, if you give those same inputs low-frequency activation for a period of several minutes, you can cause a decrease in the strength of synaptic transmission. This essentially erases the memory trace that is being stored in the neurocircuit. Memories are stored by the increase of synaptic transmission in neurocircuits, and perhaps are forgotten by the decrease in transmission in those neurocircuits. Both of these events are induced by activity that arrives at the hippocampus, either sensory activity or the lack of sensory activity.

Synapses have two parts, presynaptic and postsynaptic, that are from two separate neurons. The presynaptic neuron puts a synaptic terminal onto a postsynaptic process of another neuron, and these two neurons communicate with each other via the release of a chemical neurotransmitter—excitatory, glutamate-mediated transmission. There are several subtypes of postsynaptic glutamate receptors. One of the subtypes is an AMPA receptor, and another is a NMDA receptor. Both of these receptors are found in the postsynaptic membrane, and both are ionotropic receptors. They open the I_M channel when glutamate binds to the extra cellular binding domain. And then current will flow into the postsynaptic cell causing a synaptic current or a synaptic potential.

These two receptors differ in two important ways. First, the AMPA receptor is not voltage-dependent. That is, it will open any time glutamate binds to it, regardless of the membrane potential of the postsynaptic cell. The NMDA receptor is voltage-dependent. It will open only when the postsynaptic cell is depolarized. In fact, the NMDA receptor opens, but it is blocked by magnesium ions in a voltage-dependent way. Only if you can depolarize the postsynaptic cells efficiently, can you actually get current flow through that NMDA receptor. In summary, AMPA receptors are not voltage-dependent, and NMDA receptors are voltage-dependent.

The second important difference is that the AMPA receptor, when it carries current across the postsynaptic membrane, carries primarily sodium and potassium currents, but no calcium. The NMDA receptor, on the other hand, carries sodium, potassium, and calcium. The triggering factor for both long-term potentiation and long-term depression is the calcium that comes into the NMDA receptor. When a lot of calcium comes through the NMDA receptor the strength of the synapse increases, and, conversely when only a little calcium comes through, the strength of the synapse decreases. Finally, there is a pool of AMPA receptors, which are tethered in some intracellular compartment, which are not on the surface, and, therefore, do not detect the glutamate, which is coming from the presynaptic cell.

When you subject a cell to high-frequency stimulation, calcium is coming into the NMDA receptor. This calcium causes the untethering of the intracellular AMPA receptors, which then are inserted into the membrane. The population of AMPA receptors in the membrane is now greater. The glutamate, which is released by the presynaptic cell, now is detected more efficaciously, and the strength of the synapse is increased. That is long-term potentiation. And those AMPA receptors dwell persistently in the membrane as long as you do not take them out by some other manipulation. Conversely, if you apply low-frequency stimulation to the synapse, typically at about a rate of about 1 hertz, the AMPA receptors will then come back out of the membrane and go back to their intracellular tether, decreasing the strength of the synapse back to where it was before you potentiated it.

This is the basic mechanism of long-term potentiation and long-term depression. The reason why you get a greater calcium influx during high-frequency stimulation is simply that the AMPA receptor is activated repetitively and it summates the depolarization of the postsynaptic cell, therefore letting a lot calcium into the NMDA receptor. With one-hertz stimulation there is far less summation and far less calcium enters through the NMDA receptor, resulting in long-term depression.

In the hippocampus, a fairly large proportion of synapses are so-called silent synapses. Silent synapses are basically synapses that do not have any AMPA receptors in their postsynaptic membrane. They have AMPA receptors, but they are all tethered intracellularly. When glutamate is released by a silent synapse there is no response in the resting membrane potential of the cell because the AMPA receptor is not there, and the NMDA receptor will not pass current at the resting potential. You can see a synaptic current at a silent synapse only if you depolarize the postsynaptic cell to unblock the NMDA receptor. It is not exactly silent as it is actually releasing transmitter. It is more like it is deaf. The postsynaptic cell cannot "hear" the release of the transmitter. These silent synapses are really an important theme for the rest of this talk.

Long-term potentiation has been studied intensely for about thirty years. There were a number of questions, which have proven to be relatively intractable in terms of trying to figure out the mechanism, e.g., AMPA receptor movement, which is a fairly recent finding. But even more basic questions really were not understood. The reason why it was so difficult to answer these questions was that the techniques that were available depended on the study of large populations of synapses. When people were trying to understand I_M channel function with whole cell currents, all they could get was a broad outline of what permeabilities were and what kind of things I_M channel did. It required single-channel recording, where you could record from a few I_M channels at once, to really understand the details of biophysical mechanism.

We knew that the way to get at some of these intractable questions was to assess just a few synapses. We knew for a long time how to do this in principle, which was to record from just two neurons at once. The strategy was to do whole cell recording on just two neurons, which were connected synaptically. This way you can get down to the very minimum number of synapses that you could record at once.

For some time everybody understood that this was the way to proceed. The problem was that in the brain, even in fields that are meant to be synaptically connected, any two cells are only connected somewhere between one and 5 percent of the time. Consequently, finding these synaptic connections was quite difficult. Postdocs and graduate students are smart even before you teach them anything. If you tell them that there is a great study that is going to solve a lot of problems, but it is going to fail 99 percent of the time, they will be reluctant to conduct the experiment. I do not blame them.

We solved this problem by using a cultured hippocampus slice preparation. Hippocampal slices have been in use for a number of years. A hippocampal slice, can be kept in culture for about a week before we record from it. The organotypic slice retains all of the architecture of the hippocampus and it maintains all the appropriate connections that you see in the hippocampus, with one difference: the cells between the neurons in these organotypic slices hyperconnect, that is, they form more synapses than they should. They are appropriate synapses and they go to the right cells, but they make more connections than is usual. The advantage of this is that it increases the connection frequency between two cells to about 50 percent. So now postdocs and graduate students will actually imagine doing the experiment.

We developed this technique from the work of Dominic Muller. For this particular application we simply picked two cells in the CA-3 region of hippocampus because these make synapses with each other and we recorded from the two cells simultaneously You can put your electrodes down on any two cells, and see if are they connected, and about half the time they are.

If they are connected and if you depolarize one of the cells, it causes an action potential, and if it is synaptically connected it will cause a synaptic current to be produced in the postsynaptic cell. Now these connections are not necessarily unitary. Generally speaking, the number of synapses between one cell and another cell in this preparation is between about one and five.

Even though we are using small population of synapses, sometimes one, it is difficult to know which is which in any given experiment. We have to assume that there are a small number of multiple synapses when we do these experiments. Now, interestingly, we also found that sometimes it would appear that you did not have a connection. That if you stimulated the presynaptic cells nothing would happen in the postsynaptic cell. However, in about 40 percent of those cases, the cells were actually connected. They were connected by silent synapses.

One issue that immediately developed was to identify which synapses would be active and which would be silent. We developed a test to see whether the connections of a group of synapses were mixed—active and silent—or whether they were always all active or whether they were always all silent. Every once in a while Mother Nature does you a favor, and this is one case. There are never many mixed populations in these small numbers of synapses; they are almost either all active or all silent. This means that in experiments we could treat a group of synapses as one, which gave us a great experimental advantage.

In the hypothetical case where you have a mixture of silent synapses, those with no surface AMPA receptors, and active synapses, those with AMPA receptors in the cell membrane, the synaptic failure rates differ at different membrane potentials. Each one of these presynaptic synapses will release at some probability less than one. Recording from a group of synapses at once, you will obtain a rate, which represents the probability that all will fail at once. This happens about half the time that you stimulate.

In the case of a mixed population, only two synapses will be seeing the glutamate release at a hyperpolarized potential, but all will be seeing the glutamate release at depolarized potential. So if they are mixed, you should see a higher failure rate when the cell is hyperpolarized when you cannot see the silent synapses, and a lower failure rate at depolarized potential when you can see all the synapses. And conversely, if all the synapses are active, then the failure rate should be the same regardless of the membrane potential. The answer, as I already told you, is that the failure rates are not significantly different at depolarizing or hyperpolarized potentials. When you see an active connection, where you actually see a synaptic response, these connections are all active and there are no silent synapses hiding in there.

We can find cells with no active synapses. If you take and record from a presynaptic cell and a postsynaptic cell at the same time, and then go about stimulating the presynaptic cell with an action potential repeatedly, in about half the cases you see no response from the postsynaptic cell in trial after trial. About 40 percent of these cases are connected by silent synapses. They can be identified by depolarizing the postsynaptic cell and looking for the NMDA mediated synaptic current. We started with a connected pair of cells, but connected by nothing but silent synapses. When this is subjected to this stimulus, which potentiates the synapse, the silent synapses will be awakened and essentially potentiated.

When we put a memory-producing stimulus on a pair of cells, you can see they are responding to almost every action potential. You can convert silent synapses to active synapses by providing the proper kind of activity. As a control, in the other 60 percent of connections where you see nothing, you also see no NMDA response, and you cannot awaken them. They are not connected at all.

Synaptic connections between pyramidal cells can be made entirely of silent synapses. Long-term potentiation can be expressed via the unsilencing of these synapses. This occurs by the postsynaptic increase in AMPA sensitivity and both silent and active connections can potentiate. Earlier we thought that only silent synapses could be potentiated and that active synapses already had AMPA receptors. It turns out you can insert more AMPA receptors into an already active synapse; you can grade potentiation even in a single synapse. Moreover, we began to understand that there were three different states of the synapse: 1) the silent synapse state, 2) the active synapse state, and 3) the potentiated state. We are trying to understand how these different states are related. Long-term depression is the activity-dependent decrease in synaptic potential. We wondered whether we could see this in our pairs of connected cells. The answer is yes, we can. If you provide a synaptic connection between just two cells with low-frequency stimulation for a period of 10 minutes, you can suppress the strength of that synaptic connection in a permanent way, making long-term depression the state of the synapse. We obtained a depressed state, taking an active synaptic pair and depressing it by providing low-frequency stimulation. This is mediated by activation of the NMDA receptors.

In addition, we found that you can actually return synapses to their silent state, if you gave a longer period of low-frequency stimulation—20 minutes instead of 10 minutes—you could drive about half of the synapses back to being completely silent. There are about 125 traces in here after receiving a low-frequency stimulation without a single AMPA response in there. The NMDA response is still there, so we have not killed the synapse, it has just been silenced. Synapse silence was thought to just be a developmental step. When they first formed, synapses were silent, and then at some point became active and were then forever active. However, we have shown here that you can actually move back and forth between the active and the silent stages.

There is another form of synaptic depression called depotentiation where instead of simply depressing the synapse from baseline, you potentiate it first and then give a low-frequency stimulation, and return it back to its baseline. We raised the question: was this simply the same thing as long-term depression or was it a distinct process? We found that, in one sense, this is a distinct process because it does not depend on the NMDA receptor, as does the long-term depression.

If you apply the NMDA receptor antagonist when you try to depotentiate a synapse, it depotentiates just fine. If you apply another kind of receptor antagonist, such as the so-called metabotropic glutamate receptor, it completely blocks the depotentiation of synaptic transmission. So, at least in this sense, there are actually two forms of depression, the long-term depression and the depotentiation. One is mGluR dependent; one is NMDA dependent.

We found that even if we waited for some longer period of time before applying the low-frequency stimulation, that this depotentiation was still mGluR-dependent. Even if we waited an hour, which was about as long as we could manage in this experiment before we tried to depress the synapse, they were still mGluR-dependent. Within this time period there was no return to NMDA dependence; it was always mGluR-dependent.

We wanted to see what would happen if we came from the silent state of the synapse rather than the active state. We started with synapses which were silent, potentiated them, and then applied low-frequency stimulation. What we found was that you cannot depotentiate a previously silenced synapse; they are protected in some way from being redepressed. This does not last forever. If you wait 30 minutes, activate a silent synapse, and then apply the low-frequency stimulation, it can be depressed. They are initially protected from depotentiation and recover very quickly, and within about 5 minutes, they recover the ability to be depotentiated again.

This is interesting because silent synapses represent a reserve pool that can take input and store a memory maybe more effectively than an active synapse because they go from nothing to a very large synaptic response. It is interesting that these silent synapses, which may be preferentially storing new information, protect that information from low-frequency stimulation, which is impinging on neurons all the time. This leads to the suggestion that a new memory trace may be protected in some way for at least some period of time over half an hour, which, interestingly enough, is sort of the time period over which memory consolidation is thought to occur.

We knew that this recently silent state, which was protected from depression, was transitioning probably somewhere else in the model. But we did not know where to draw the line: was it a potentiated synapse at this point, or was it an active synapse? Where was the point were it recovered its ability to be depotentiated? We tested for that by looking at the receptor dependency of this recovered depotentiation.

The answer is that the recovered depotentiation of a recently silenced synapse, unlike normal depotentiation, is actually NMDA dependent, and not mGluR dependent. In addition, the other thing to recall is that if you depotentiate, it does not recover its NMDA dependence even after an hour. However, if you depotentiate an active synapse and we know that this depotentiation is mGluR dependent, it immediately switches back to being an NMDA dependent in terms of any further depression. So basically, we know that any time you can return to this active state, that any depression out of that active state is an NMDA dependent. From those two pieces of data we conclude that the vector from recently silent actually goes to active. We have these different states of the synapse: silent, depressed, active, potentiated, and their interrelationships.

Our working model is that active synapses have both NMDA and AMPA receptors, and they can potentiate, where they insert AMPA receptors into the membrane. The depotentiation from that state is now mGluR dependent, even though depression from this state is totally NMDA dependent. It raises an interesting possibility that you may be inserting not only AMPA receptors in this case, but also metabotropic glutamate receptors. Silent synapses have no AMPA receptors in their membrane, and when they are potentiated they receive AMPA receptors, but then they transition back into this active state. They are protected from any kind of depression for the first half an hour of their new life.

It is important because we know now that we can transition from this active state back to the silent state, which means you can potentially regenerate the silent synapses during the normal activity that the brain undergoes during both frequency activation or during forgetting. This sort of reloads the brain to store new memories, which can then be initially protected when new information comes in and causes a high-frequency activation of the inputs. We also know that the NMDA receptors are also regulated, which produces a kind of metaplasticity of the whole system.

The main conclusion that we have from this research is that both active and silent synapses can potentiate and that long-term potentiation can be graded in a single synapse. So all synapses are basically capable of storing memory traces; but silent synapses do it a little bit better. The synapses can exist in different states of plasticity and how they behave depends on what state they are coming from. The synapses move between these states in an activity-dependent manner, and the history of the synapse actually matters for plasticity, and therefore should matter for the way that memory traces are formed.

In closing I want to give credit where credit is due. Much of this research emerged from my laboratory and Johanna Montgomery played a prominent role in the study.

Transcription, Chromatin Assembly, and Homologous Recombination in Chromatin

James T. Kadonaga, Ph.D.
University of California, San Diego

Figure 1 is a picture that I downloaded from the human genome web site. It reflects the considerable effort that is devoted to the study of our genetic material, DNA. However, DNA in the eukaryotic nucleus is not this simple fiber, but instead is packaged into a nucleoprotein complex termed chromatin.

Figure 2 is an electron micrograph of chromatin. This picture displays the periodic nature of chromatin, as the unfolded chromatin filament resembles beads on a string. Figure 3 shows a schematic diagram of chromatin. The DNA (in black) is wound around the core histones in yellow. The linker histone H1 is shown in blue.

The monomeric unit of this repeated structure is called the nucleosome. Figure 4 shows the x-ray crystal structure of the nucleosome, which was solved by Tim Richmond and coworkers a few years ago. It depicts the nice balance between the DNA and the histones. In native chromatin, the DNA to protein mass ratio is approximately 1 to 1. So, it is probably most reasonable to think that the DNA and histones act as partners, rather than as one dominant over the other.

What happens in chromatin? Basically, whatever happens in DNA, happens in chromatin (Figure 5). Here we have things like transcription and DNA replication, repair, and recombination. But there are also chromatin-specific processes, such as chromatin assembly and the post-translational modification of histones. In addition, there is euchromatin in which most transcribed genes are located as well as heterochromatin, which includes centromeres and telomeres.

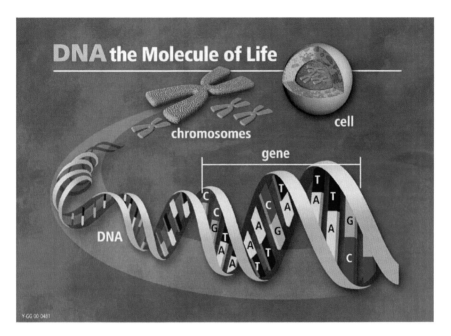

FIGURE 1 DNA—the molecule of life.
SOURCE: http://www.ornl.gov/TechResources/Human_Genome/

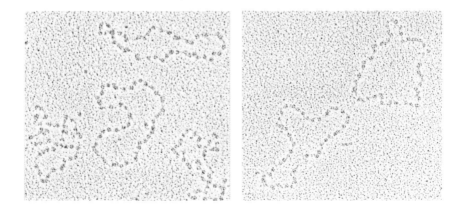

FIGURE 2 Eukaryotic DNA package into chromatin.

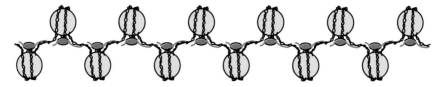

FIGURE 3 Schematic diagram of the 10 nm diameter chromatin fiber.

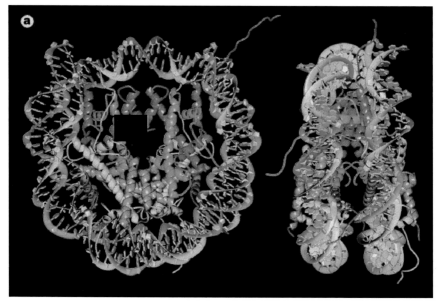

FIGURE 4 Crystal structure of the Nucleosome.
SOURCE: Luger, K., Mäder, A. W., Richmond, R. K., Sargent, D. F., and Richmond, T. J. (1997). Crystal structure of the nucleosome core particle at 2.8 Å resolution. *Nature* 389:251-260.

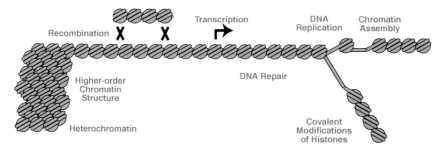

FIGURE 5 A variety of biological phenomena involve chromatin.

I am going to give you three short stories that describe some of the things that we do in my lab. The first story actually does not involve chromatin itself, but instead focuses on the basic transcription process. Second, I am going to talk about chromatin assembly, and then lastly, I am going to say a few words on homologous recombination in chromatin.

TRANSCRIPTION

Figure 6 is from before I used computers to make graphics. What we have here is a typical eukaryotic transcriptional control region. In our genome, we have several tens of thousands of genes, and each one has its own unique transcriptional program. Now, we are faced with the challenge of understanding how the activity of each of these tens of thousands of genes is regulated. One approach to this problem is the analysis of the fundamental mechanisms by which transcription is regulated—and that is the general question that we address.

One key DNA element that is involved in transcription is the core promoter, which contains the information that is needed for the RNA polymerase II transcriptional machinery to initiate transcription. The core promoter is typically about 40 bp in length and encompasses the transcription start site.

Immediately upstream of the core promoter, there is the proximal promoter region. In this region, there are recognition sites for sequence-specific DNA binding transcription factors, such as Sp1. Then, at variable distances from the core promoter—which could be either upstream or downstream of the start site—are transcriptional enhancers. Enhancers typically contain many recognition sites for the binding of a wide variety of sequence-specific DNA binding factors, and can be located as far as 80 kbp from the core promoter.

Figure 7 is a modernized version of Figure 6. Things have gotten more complicated over the years, but we still have the DNA, the core promoter, and the promoter- and enhancer-binding factors. And now, we also have nucleosomes in the picture. In addition, there are coactivators

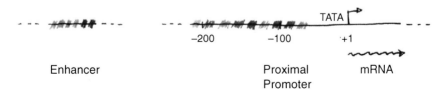

FIGURE 6 A typical Eukaryotic transcription control region.

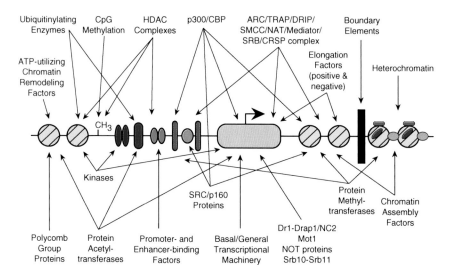

FIGURE 7 Many factors affect the regulation of transcription by RNA polymerase II.

that link the activators to the basal machinery as well as all sorts of histone-modifying enzymes and nucleosome-mobilizing factors. So, it is a fairly complicated picture.

I am going talk about the core promoter—just what is happening at the RNA start site, and why would anybody ever want to study that? I think that it is important to know how the basic transcription process works in eukaryotes. And second, when you look at the function of all of these factors (shown in Figure 7)—all of these coactivators, coregulators, histone-modifying enzymes, and nucleosome-remodeling factors—after they are done doing what they do, the transcriptional signals ultimately lead to the core promoter. In other words, all transcriptional pathways ultimately lead to the core promoter. Thus, the core promoter is the ultimate target of all of the factors that regulate the initiation of gene transcription.

Today, I am going to focus on the cis-acting DNA elements in the core promoter (Figure 8). Most of you are probably familiar with the TATA box motif that is located about 25-30 nucleotides upstream of the transcription start site. The TATA box is, by far, the most widely studied core promoter motif, and it is sometimes incorrectly thought that all core promoters contain a TATA box. But, in humans, it is estimated that perhaps only about 30 percent of core promoters have a TATA box. It then follows

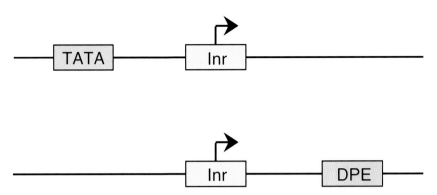

FIGURE 8 TATA versus DPE-dependent core promoters.

that about 70 percent of core promoters in humans do not have a TATA. We therefore felt that it would be important to understand the core promoter elements that are involved in the transcription of the large proportion of genes that lack a TATA box.

These studies led Tom Burke to the discovery of a downstream core promoter motif called the DPE, which is located about 30 nucleotides downstream of the transcription start site. The DPE is conserved from *Drosophila* to humans, and is most commonly found in TATA-less promoters. In DPE-dependent promoters, the spacing between the DPE and Initiator (Inr) motifs appears to be invariant. Like the TATA box, the DPE is a sequence-specific recognition site for the TFIID basal transcription factor, which binds cooperatively to the Inr and DPE motifs. Also, if you inactivate a TATA-dependent promoter by mutation of the TATA box, you can restore the activity of the core promoter by the addition of a DPE motif at its appropriate downstream location.

How common is the DPE? Alan Kutach carried out a statistical analysis of about 200 core promoters in *Drosophila* and found that about 29 percent of the promoters have a TATA box and no DPE, about 26 percent have a DPE and no TATA, about 14 percent have both, and about 31 percent have neither a TATA nor a DPE (Figure 9). So, it appears that the DPE is about as common as the TATA box in *Drosophila*.

It seemed possible that the fundamental mechanism of basal transcription from TATA-dependent promoters is different from the mechanism of transcription from DPE-dependent promoters. In fact, that appears to be the case. For instance, Trish Willy identified and purified an activity that activates DPE transcription but not TATA transcription, and found that this activity is mediated by a protein termed NC2 (Dr1-Drap1)

Promoter Type

**Occurrence in Natural
Drosophila Promoters**

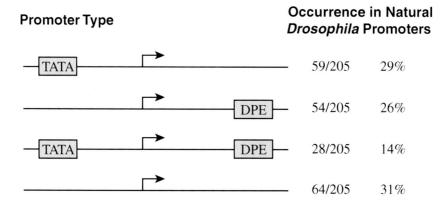

TATA →	59/205	29%
→ DPE	54/205	26%
TATA → DPE	28/205	14%
→	64/205	31%

FIGURE 9 Frequency of occurrence of TATA box and DPE motifs in *Drosophila* core promoters.
SOURCE: Kutach, A. K., and Kadonaga, J. T. (2000). The downstream promoter element DPE appears to be as widely used as the TATA box in *Drosophila* core promoters. *Mol. Cell. Biol.* 20:4754-4764. Fig. 4A.

(Figure 10). NC2 (Dr1-Drap1) was initially purified by several labs as a repressor of TATA transcription. What Trish found is that it is an activator of DPE transcription. Thus, NC2 (Dr1-Drap1) is a factor that can discriminate between TATA- versus DPE-dependent core promoters. Moreover, Trish identified a mutant form of NC2 (Dr1-Drap1) that is able to activate DPE transcription but unable to repress TATA transcription. This result indicates that the activation of DPE-dependent transcription by NC2 (Dr1-Drap1) is distinct from its repression of TATA-dependent transcription. Trish's findings exemplify the differences in the basic mechanisms of transcription from DPE-dependent versus TATA-dependent core promoters.

One other question that we asked was—why would a gene have a DPE or a TATA box in its core promoter? One somewhat fanciful idea was that the presence of a TATA or DPE motif might be important for the proper functioning of some transcriptional enhancers. As shown in Figure 11, sometimes you have a cluster of genes in which the yellow enhancer needs to find the yellow promoter, the blue enhancer needs to find the blue promoter, and so on. Enhancer-core promoter interactions may be one means by which such enhancer-promoter specificity is achieved.

To test this idea, Jenny Butler used a *Drosophila* P-element transformation construct called the waffle vector Figure 12. She inserted two related reporter genes into the waffle vector: DPE-*GFP* and TATA-*GFP*. DPE-*GFP* has a DPE-dependent core promoter, and TATA-*GFP* has a

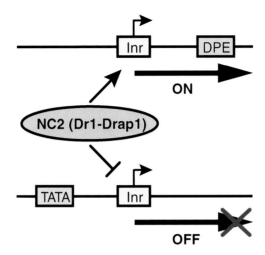

FIGURE 10 NC2 (Dr1-Drap1) is a bifuncational, core-pomoter-specific transcription factor.
SOURCE: Willy, P. J., Kobayashi, R., and Kadonaga, J. T. (2000). A basal transcription factor that activates or represses transcription. *Science* 290:982-984. Fig. 4B.

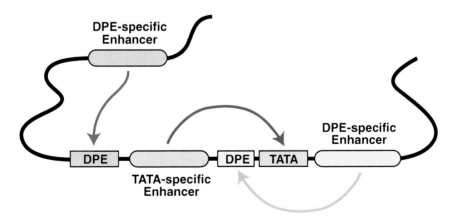

FIGURE 11 TATA or DPE motif might be important for the proper functioning of some transcriptional enhancers.
SOURCE: Butler, J. E. F., and Kadonaga, J. T. (2001). Enhancer-promoter specificity mediated by DPE or TATA core promoter motifs. *Genes Dev.* 15:2515-2519. Fig. 1.

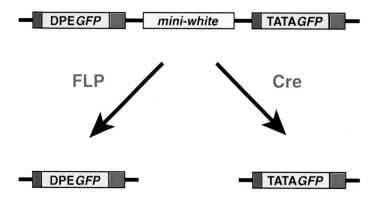

FIGURE 12 The waffle vectorgeneates allelic transgenes.

TATA-dependent core promoter. These two genes are identical except for seven nucleotides in the TATA box region and seven nucleotides at the DPE region. Jenny transformed flies with her waffle construct, and then used enhancer-trapping techniques to mobilize the element transiently. The biallelic construct would occasionally land near an enhancer, which would activate transcription from either or both of the reporter genes. To compare the effect of each trapped enhancer upon transcription from DPE-*GFP* relative to that from TATA-*GFP*, Jenny created two daughter lines by the use of either FLP recombinase (in blue) or Cre recombinase (in red) in vivo. As shown at the bottom of Figure 12, this procedure results in the generation of two sister lines that have chromosomes that are identical except for the 14 nucleotides at the TATA and DPE regions of the core promoter. In this manner, Jenny was able to determine the effect of randomly-trapped enhancers upon DPE-versus TATA-dependent transcription.

These experiments showed that there are indeed DPE- and TATA-specific transcriptional enhancers Figure 13. Approximately 25 percent of the enhancers that we tested exhibit specificity for the TATA or DPE motifs. Thus, some enhancers function specifically with DPE or TATA elements in the core promoter. More generally, these results indicate that the core promoter is much more than a sequence that directs the proper site of initiation by RNA polymerase II. Rather, the core promoter is an important regulatory element.

A corollary to these conclusions is that if you are studying your favorite enhancer, you should do it in conjunction with its cognate core promoter. It is a common practice to map enhancers by fusing portions of the

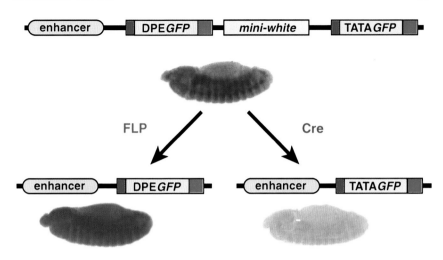

FIGURE 13 Identification of a DPE-specific enhancer.
SOURCE: Butler, J. E. F., and Kadonaga, J. T. (2001). Enhancer-promoter specificity mediated by DPE or TATA core promoter motifs. *Genes Dev.* 15:2515-2519. Fig. 3B.

enhancer region with a generic TATA-containing reporter gene. In such an assay, a DPE-specific enhancer would not be detected.

To summarize the studies of the core promoter—we have identified and characterized a new core promoter motif termed the DPE (Figure 8). The DPE is a downstream core promoter element that is located around +30 relative to the transcription start site. The DPE is conserved from *Drosophila* to humans, and is a binding site for TFIID. In *Drosophila*, the DPE is about as common as the TATA box. We found that NC2 (Dr1-Drap1), which had been previously studied as a repressor of transcription from TATA-dependent promoters, is an activator of transcription from DPE-dependent promoters. We have also found that the presence of a DPE or TATA motif in the core promoter can have a critical role in enhancer function.

CHROMATIN ASSEMBLY

Next, I will describe some of our studies in the area of chromatin assembly. So, why would anybody want to study chromatin assembly? In eukaryotes, genome replication is really chromosome replication, and chromosome replication requires the duplication of the DNA and the assembly of the newly-replicated DNA into chromatin. In fact, chromatin assembly is required whenever DNA is synthesized, such as during repli-

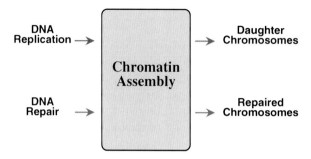

FIGURE 14 Chromatin assembly is important for chromosome structure.

cation or repair. In Figure 14 I have depicted chromatin assembly as something of a "light blue box" rather than a "black box."

Our studies of chromatin assembly began with the development of a
crude *Drosophila* embryo extract, termed the S-190 that mediates the ATP-
dependent assembly of periodic nucleosome arrays. This was the work of
Rohinton Kamakaka and Mike Bulger. (I should point out here that Abe
Worcel, in the early 1980s, pioneered the development of an ATP-dependent chromatin assembly extract from *Xenopus* oocytes.) Our *Drosophila* S-
190 extract was designed, in particular, to be scaled up for the subsequent
fractionation and purification of the assembly factors. To this end, Mike
Bulger, Takashi Ito, and Jessica Tyler had fractionated, purified, and
cloned the factors that mediate the ATP-dependent assembly of periodic
nucleosome arrays. These studies led to the discovery of the ATP-utiliz-
ing motor protein involved in chromatin assembly, which is termed ACF,
as well as one novel histone chaperone, ASF1, and three previously-
known histone chaperones, CAF-1, NAP-1, and nucleoplasmin (Figure
15). ACF is the source of the ATP-dependence of the chromatin assembly
reaction, and it is needed for both histone deposition and periodic nucleosome spacing. ACF comprises the ISWI ATPase motor and an Acf1 large
subunit, which appears to 'program' the ISWI motor. Chromatin assembly can be mediated by ACF in conjunction with a core histone chaperone.

Today, we now have a completely purified, recombinant system for
the ATP-dependent assembly of periodic nucleosome arrays (Figure 16).
This system was developed by Dmitry Fyodorov and Mark Levenstein. It
consists of purified recombinant ACF, purified recombinant NAP-1 (as
the histone chaperone), purified native (or recombinant) core histones,
DNA, and ATP.

We typically monitor the assembly of chromatin by using the micrococcal nuclease digestion assay (Figure 17). In this assay, chromatin is

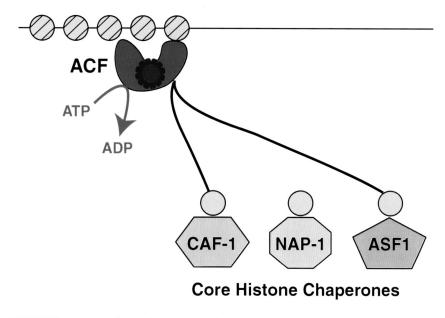

FIGURE 15 A simple working model for chromatin assembly.

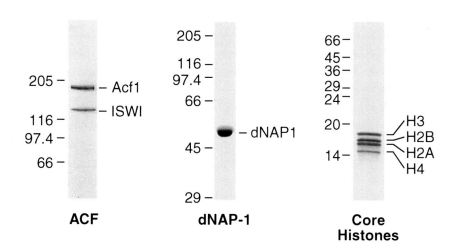

FIGURE 16 Purified chromatin assembly factor and core histones.
SOURCE: Jiang, W., Nordeen, S. K., and Kadonaga, J. T. (2000). Transcriptional analysis of chromatin assembled with purified ACF and dNAP1 reveals that acetyl CoA is required for preinitiation complex assembly. *J. Biol. Chem.* 275: 39819-39822. Fig. 1.

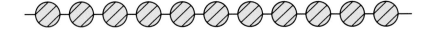

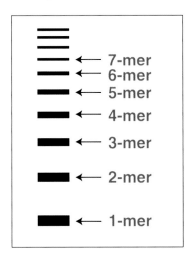

FIGURE 17 Micrococcal nucleas digestion assay.
SOURCE: Ito, T., Levenstein, M. E., Fyodorov, D. V., Kutach, A. K., Kobayashi, R., and Kadonaga, J. T. (1999). ACF consists of two subunits, Acf1 and ISWI, that function cooperatively in the ATP-dependent catalysis of chromatin assembly. *Genes Dev.* 13:1529-1539. Fig. 4C.

partially digested with micrococcal nuclease, which makes a double-stranded cleavage in the linker DNA between the nucleosomes. Then, the oligonucleosomal fragments are deproteinized, and the resulting DNAs are resolved by agarose gel electrophoresis. If you have a periodic nucleosome array, then the DNA fragments derived from each oligonucleosome population (i.e., 1-mers, 2-mers, 3-mers, 4-mers, etc.) would each be of approximately the same length, and a DNA "ladder" would be obtained.

When we assemble chromatin with our purified factors and analyze the products by the micrococcal nuclease digestion assay, we see that there is efficient assembly of periodic nucleosome arrays (Figure 18). Each protomer of ACF can assemble at least 50 nucleosomes.

To study how ACF works, Dmitry Fyodorov performed template-commitment experiments as well as other related mechanistic analyses. His results suggest that ACF is a processive, ATP-driven motor that trans-locates along DNA and mediates chromatin assembly (Figure 19). Dmitry also carried out a genetic analysis of ACF in vivo in *Drosophila*. These studies have revealed that ACF influences the cell cycle as well as gene expression.

To summarize this section on chromatin assembly—we have fractionated, purified, and cloned the factors that mediate chromatin assembly. These studies led, in particular, to the discovery of ACF. In this work, we have achieved a purified, recombinant chromatin assembly system with ACF and dNAP1. The only other factors needed are core histones, DNA, and ATP. We have also found that ACF appears to function as a processive, ATP-driven motor that assembles nucleosomes as it translocates along DNA.

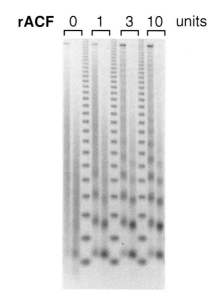

[1 unit corresponds to an
ACF:octamer ratio of 1:150]

FIGURE 18 Chromatin assembly with purified, recombinant ACF.

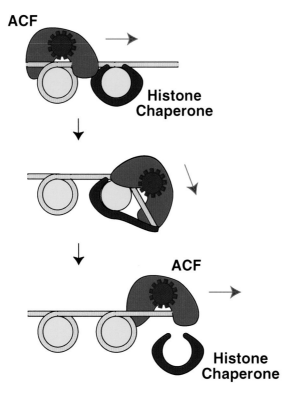

FIGURE 19 A processive model for chromatin assembly.

HOMOLOGOUS RECOMBINATION IN CHROMATIN

Lastly, I will describe some of our studies of homologous recombination in chromatin. This work was carried out by Vassili Alexiadis. These experiments were inspired by two things—first, homologous recombination is a fundamental and important biological process; and second, the Rad54 protein, which is involved in homologous recombination, is a member of the Snf2-like family of ATPases, which comprises the ATPase subunits of all known chromatin remodeling complexes (Figure 20). For instance, Rad54 is related to the ISWI ATPase subunit of ACF. Thus, it seemed likely that Rad54 would have a chromatin-related function in homologous recombination.

Rad54 is involved in homologous recombination during double-strand break repair as well as during meiosis. Rad54 and Rad51, which is related to bacterial RecA protein, participate in the strand pairing reaction that yields a D loop (Figure 21).

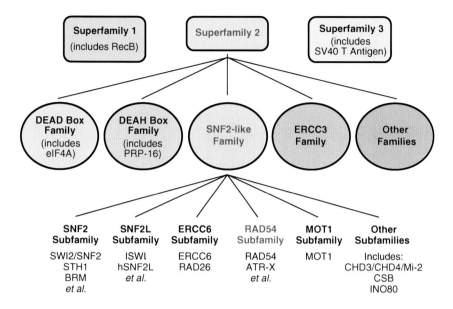

FIGURE 20 Helicases and related protein with conserved NTP-binding mofits. SOURCE: Corbalenya, A. E., and Koonin, E. V., *Curr. Opin. Struct. Biol.* 3:419-429 (1993). Eisen et al., *Nucleic Acids Res.* 23:2715-2723 (1995).

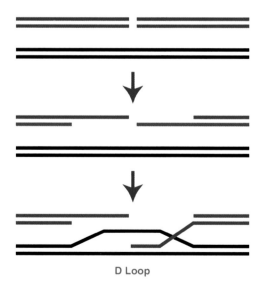

D Loop

FIGURE 21 Initial steps of homologous recombination at a double-strand break.

There are different ways by which this strand pairing reaction can be carried out in vitro. Vassili used an assay with double-stranded circular plasmid DNA and a homologous single-stranded oligonucleotide (Figure 22). In this reaction, Rad51 associates with the single-stranded oligonucleotide in an ATP-dependent manner, and then forms a D loop in a reaction that requires Rad54 and ATP. When he carries out this reaction with purified Rad54 and Rad51, he observes that the formation of D loops requires Rad51, Rad54, ATP, and homologous single-stranded DNA (Figure 23).

Next, Vassili sought to use chromatin instead of DNA in these reactions (Figure 24). These experiments revealed that Rad54 and Rad51 work at least as well with chromatin as with naked DNA (Figure 25). In contrast, the bacterial RecA protein can catalyze D loop formation with naked DNA but not with chromatin. Thus, Rad54 and Rad51 work well in chromatin.

Vassili then sought to investigate the effect of superhelical tension upon D loop formation by Rad51 and Rad54, because the bulk of the eukaryotic genome possesses little superhelical tension. He therefore tested the effect of relaxation of superhelical tension upon D loop formation by Rad51 and Rad54. These experiments revealed that relaxation of naked DNA by topoisomerase I results in a greater than 100-fold decrease

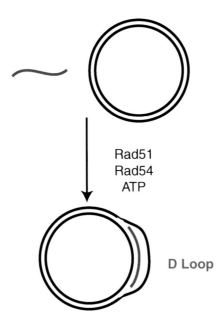

FIGURE 22 Catalysis of strand pairing by Rad51 and Rad54.

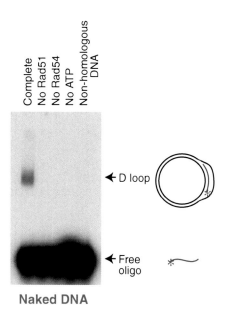

Naked DNA

FIGURE 23 Formation of D loops with purified Rad51 and Rad54.
SOURCE: Alexiadis, V., and Kadonaga, J. T. (2002). Strand pairing by Rad54 and Rad51 is enhanced by chromatin. *Genes Dev.* 16:2767-2771. Fig. 1B.

in D loop formation by Rad54 and Rad51. In constrast, he found that topoisomerase I-mediated relaxation of chromatin has no effect upon the efficiency of D loop formation by Rad51 and Rad54 (Figure 26). Thus, the packaging of DNA into chromatin facilitates D loop formation by over 100-fold in the absence of superhelical tension.

To test further whether chromatin is important for D loop formation by Rad54 and Rad51, Vassili employed a different experimental approach. Instead of relaxing preassembled chromatin, he assembled relaxed DNA into chromatin and then performed D loop reactions. To this end, he assembled relaxed DNA into chromatin by using purified recombinant ACF, purified recombinant NAP-1, purified core histones, relaxed plasmid DNA, and ATP in the presence of purified topoisomerase I. These reactions were performed in the absence (no chromatin assembly) or presence (chromatin assembly) of core histones. As seen in this slide (Figure 27), the packaging of relaxed DNA into chromatin results in a greater than 100-fold stimulation of D loop formation by Rad54 and Rad51.

Hence, Rad51 and Rad54, but not *E. coli* RecA, can form D loops with chromatin. Notably, there is a greater than 100-fold enhancement of strand pairing by Rad54 and Rad51 upon assembly of relaxed DNA into chroma-

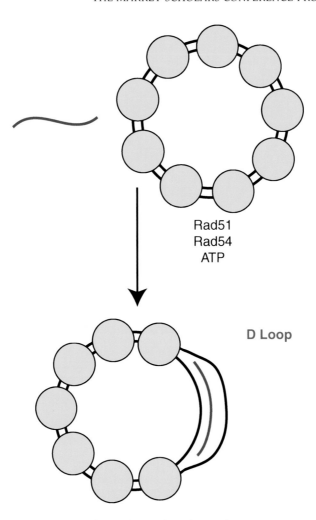

FIGURE 24 Strand pairing by Rad51 and Rad54 in chromatin.

tin. We have also found that Rad54 and Rad51 function cooperatively in the ATP-dependent remodeling of chromatin. It is generally thought that chromatin represses DNA-directed processes, such as transcription and replication, but here we have an example of a DNA-utilizing process that is *facilitated* by the packaging of DNA into chromatin. These results indicate that Rad54 and Rad51 have evolved to function optimally with chromatin (Figure 28). In addition, these findings may be applicable to studies of homologous recombination in vivo, such as for targeted knockouts and gene therapy.

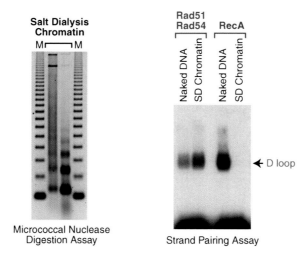

FIGURE 25 Rad51 and Rad54, but not RecA, can form D loops with chromatin.
SOURCE: Alexiadis, V., and Kadonaga, J. T. (2002). Strand pairing by Rad54 and
Rad51 is enhanced by chromatin. *Genes Dev.* 16:2767-2771. Fig. 2B.

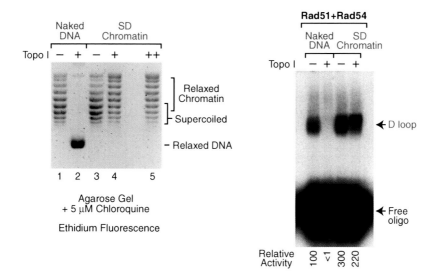

FIGURE 26 Chromatin facilitates D loop formation in the absence of superhelical
tension.
SOURCE: Alexiadis, V., and Kadonaga, J. T. (2002). Strand pairing by Rad54 and
Rad51 is enhanced by chromatin. *Genes Dev.* 16:2767-2771. Fig. 3.

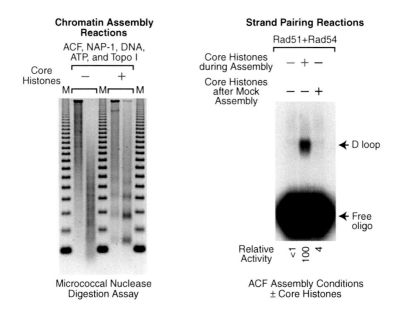

FIGURE 27 The assembly of relaxed DNA into chromatin facilitates strand pairing by Rad54 and Rad51.

SOURCE: Alexiadis, V., and Kadonaga, J. T. (2002). Strand pairing by Rad54 and Rad51 is enhanced by chromatin. *Genes Dev.* 16:2767-2771. Fig. 4.

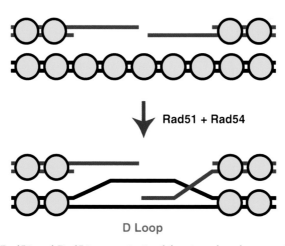

FIGURE 28 Rad51 and Rad54 are optimized for strand exchange with chromatin.

SUMMARY

To summarize—I have described some of our studies in the area of basal transcription, chromatin assembly, and homologous recombination. In the area of basal transcription, we have identified and characterized the DPE downstream core promoter motif. The DPE is conserved from *Drosophila* to humans, and is something of a downstream analogue of the TATA box. Notably, some transcriptional enhancers act specifically with core promoters that contain a DPE or TATA motif. Thus, the core promoter can be an important component in the regulation of a gene.

In the area of chromatin assembly, we have fractionated, purified, and cloned the factors that mediate the ATP-dependent assembly of periodic nucleosome arrays. These studies led, in particular, to the discovery of ACF. In this work, we have achieved a purified, recombinant chromatin assembly system with ACF, NAP-1, core histones, DNA, and ATP. Mechanistic studies suggest that ACF functions as a processive, ATP-driven motor that translocates along DNA and mediates chromatin assembly.

We have also investigated the role of chromatin in homologous recombination in vitro. We observed a greater than 100-fold enhancement of strand pairing by Rad54 and Rad51 with chromatin in the absence of superhelical tension. In addition, we found that Rad54 and Rad51 function cooperatively in the remodeling of chromatin. These results indicate that Rad54 and Rad51 have evolved to function with chromatin, the natural substrate, rather than with naked DNA.

Lastly, and most importantly, I would like to mention the past and present coworkers who have contributed to this work (Figure 29). Tom Burke discovered the DPE, Alan Kutach studied the DPE consensus sequence, Trish Willy identified NC2 (Dr1-Drap1) as an activator of DPE-dependent but not TATA-dependent transcription, and Jenny Butler identified the DPE-specific transcriptional enhancers. Rohinton Kamakaka and Mike Bulger developed the S-190 chromatin assembly extract, Mike Bulger and Takashi Ito performed the fractionation of the S-190 and the purification of ACF, Jessica Tyler identified and purified the ASF1/RCAF assembly factor, Dmitry Fyodorov and Mark Levenstein established the purified recombinant chromatin assembly system, and Dmitry carried out the experiments suggesting that ACF is a processive DNA-translocating enzyme as well as the genetic analysis of ACF. Vassili Alexiadis performed the studies of homologous recombination with Rad54 and Rad51 in chromatin.

DPE

Tom Burke
Alan Kutach
Patricia Willy
Jenny Butler
Tammy Juven-Gershon
Tom Boulay
Chin Yan Lim
Emily Dong

Protein biochemistry

Ryuji Kobayashi (MD Anderson)

ACF

Rohinton Kamakaka
Mike Bulger
Takashi Ito
Jessica Tyler
Mark Levenstein
Dmitry Fyodorov
Karl Haushalter

Rad54

Vassili Alexiadis

Section of Molecular Biology
UC San Diego

FIGURE 29 Coworkers and collaborators (past and present).

The New Biology

David C. Schwartz, Ph.D.
University of Wisconsin

I was contacted by Jim Kadonaga and asked to take a look into the future and describe what I saw at that edge—for which I call, "The New Biology." I believe right now that biology is in the midst of a major paradigm shift, and I think a lot of it is due to advances in information technology and the new systems that provide huge experimental data sets. Information technology is going to enhance the way that we do science in many ways, giving opportunities and challenges to a broad range of scientists, engineers, and mathematicians.

The New Biology has the three following components. It is about one third statistics, mathematics, and computer science. Another third is more in the physical sciences—physics, chemistry, and engineering. Finally, the balance is in the biological sciences and genetics. Different people will be attracted to different components and a major challenge at the university level is how to train young researchers to become the New Biologists.

The New Biologist must be able to commingle these different disciplines to address important biological problems. Teamwork is necessary since the systems that you are dealing with are very complex, and beyond the ability of an individual, or even a small laboratory to fully encompass. Some of these systems may involve complex instrumentation, but the level of complexity goes beyond instrumentation.

The fundamental nature of the systems we scientists deal with has entirely changed, and when I speak of systems, I do not mean instrumentation. I am going to talk about the very stuff that you put your fingers on, the very data that you look at, and especially the very phenomena you use to interrogate your biological systems. Let me give you some examples of advances in the New Biology.

- We are all comfortable thinking about genes. Now, we are accustomed to thinking about many genes, and lately we think about whole genomes—not only one genome, but many genomes that span populations and species. Look at the databases, and you will see hundreds of microbial genome sequences—and this is just the beginning.
- We are used to dealing with many cells. Now we can deal with single cells, in a new way, with the intent of building capacious ensembles from complex measurements obtained from a large number of individually interrogated cells. The goal is to be able to perform sophisticated experiments within a single cell and to acquire data sets that encompass large cell populations, which simultaneously require and potentiate statistical interpretation. In other words, new approaches allow us to massively "test tube-ize" cells.
- Being able to do science with single molecules has become a very popular coin of the realm. It is not difficult, and it gives you a great deal of power in terms of forming your ensembles and represents the ultimate in the ongoing quest for ever-increasing levels of miniaturization.
- We are going from instruments that used to occupy a lot of lab space to chip-based instruments that can create labs on a chip. Here, we have scaled down large instruments to reside on a single chip. In this regard, what I urge people to do is if you are going to miniaturize, revel in the scale of matter that you are working in. Take advantage of the novel phenomena that this scale gives you. It is proven to be a very interesting problem in its own right in terms of great nanotechnology and physics.
- Achieving sub-Dalton resolution, means utilizing mass spectroscopy—it is just amazing what you can do with mass spectroscopy. When I was in graduate school in chemistry, I had friends working in mass spectrometry. One day, after too many beers, someone wondered what would happen if you put a protein in a mass spectrometer. Everyone had a good laugh. Nobody is laughing anymore.
- Now the best label is no label. So we are going from labeling substrates to not labeling, yet maintaining the ability to detect with some specificity; for example surface plasmon resonance approaches offer this advantage—my Wisconsin colleagues boast about the fact that they could do chips and other types of assays with no labels, thus enabling biomolecules to function in a more native environment.
- When I was in graduate school we were able to create a limited number of compounds and characterize them. Now, combinatorial chemical libraries hold tens of thousands of characterized compounds that can be further "functionalized" through series of biological assays.

I think the modes of inquiry have changed. We are used to hearing about discovery-based science using large-scale screens. This approach leverages chance resulting from the ability to cast a large experimental net. Earlier, we heard about the fantastic work that Regeneron is doing in this area from George Yancopoulos. Discovery is the ability to do large-scale screens that produce useful information. I dare say that we are not as smart as we think we are, so being able to toss the dice in a very systematic and controlled way helps us solve very tough scientific problems.

We are trained as scientists to do hypothesis-driven research. But we can go beyond this when we blend discovery with hypothesis. Chance favors the prepared mind—I think that is a quote from Louis Pasteur, who was an accomplished chemist as well as a pioneering microbiologist. In the New Biology, the ultimate experimental space is a single molecule, or a single cell, or a single-molecule system rapidly analyzed at high resolution over a large population. At the end of the day you want to nimbly create large multidimensional databases that directly help you solve problems that are biologically relevant. With all of this data, you are not going to analyze this on a spreadsheet, so the need for sophisticated statistical and computational approaches becomes acute.

Given large data sets has encouraged many of us to become very friendly with our local computer scientists, statisticians, and even mathematicians. And while it is interesting explaining our systems to these people, it is becoming a thing of the past. Are we faced with a problem of too much information? No, I do not think so. Instead, I think that we are suffering from too little information. We have enough information to tell us what we do not know. We have enough information to tease us; but we do not have enough information to close many stories. I think that we need to find new ways to augment and balance large-scale experimental design and analysis. Given the new experimental approaches and databases that we have, are we generating the type of experiments that make sense of these data?

When I say "sense of these data" I am describing chip data, for one example. Researchers want to make sense of expression profiles. In many cases, the interesting features in a complex dataset are going to be buried deep within the data and obscured by noise, and, consequently, may not be represented at all. Subsequent activities center on slow "conventional" ad hoc experimentation and analysis to confirm "results" and then the drilling down into a select group of candidates to do proper scientific investigation with the intent of making a story. Such activities usually require several graduate/postdoc years per candidate. So the idea is to design new experimental systems that intrinsically work with operations in cyberspace—you want systems that are designed to rapidly close stories on a large number of candidates. This all begs the question, "can massive candidate identification be adequately addressed experimentally?"

Let's talk about theory and experiment. As a biologist you have ideas and you have hypotheses. But just having an idea and a hypothesis is never sufficient; you need to do experiments. So you utilize experimental spaces available to the New Biologist:

- sequence from an ABI-3700,
- large databases with other scientists' data,
- chip data,
- mass spectroscopy,
- and, if you have a lot of money, utilization of a sequencing center.

What happens is that you wind up in a loop. You come up with an idea, and may go to the databases; ultimately you sit in front of your computer. You might do some simulations, and then you come up with some candidates. And you might stay within this space a bit to refine what candidates you have. And you had better, because when you get down to the experimental end, things start slowing down a whole lot.

When I do one experiment, it seems to beget a lot more experiments. I tend to root into a problem; I get new ideas; I interact with the experimental matter: and I want to do more experiments. This process can get very slow. One solution is to have large, automated systems, enabling you to come up with even more experimental candidates that will keep a thousand postdocs busy. The loop starts out very quickly and then slows down. What is the problem; how do we expedite this loop that covers hypothesis generation and validation through experiments? We need to dramatically accelerate our ability to create and analyze complex experiments within the context of hypothesis generation.

I am a big fan of large, complex datasets. I have been using Bayesian inference techniques to analyze data. Not being a computer scientist or statistician, I am absolutely in awe of this technique. You define your system in terms of models, that describe your experimental variables, and errors—add to this a large experimental data set and then exhaustive analysis enables you to determine the best fit between your data and the "best" answer. The necessary component of this process is the availability of a large and sometimes complex dataset; obviously this approach will not solve all problems.

Let's take a look at how physicists deal with theory and experiment. Particle physicists work at very high energies, and their "city-sized" experiments produce incredibly large data sets that establish their functional loop between hypothesis and empirical data. At the European Organization for Nuclear Research (CERN) there is a cyclotron ring that is about 27 kilometers across. One experimental system at CERN handles as much information as the entire European telecommunications network does today—about 800 million-proton collisions a second, and they are able to cull from such data very rare events. They detect something of interest in one out of every hundred million, million collisions. If we were to equate this to something more biological, and this is not a perfect analogy, it means that the human genome dataset could be decoded in seconds, and lately we can envision systems that might be able to do this. Evaluating screens for point mutations means finding one mutation in a genome that is 30,000 times larger than the human genome; however, beautifully designed genetic screens can be designed for specific criteria, which similarly scale. Overall, these vignettes and comparisons provide some context on how far biological research needs to advance in terms of the generation and analysis of large datasets. In this regard, I think our problems will prove to be more difficult to solve.

We are talking then about the hard problem of generating large biologically relevant datasets and at the same time making scientific sense out of the results that come from these efforts. Up to now, we have largely relied on automation and multiplexing to do the experimental heavy lifting, and at times these activities are walled off from our hypothesis and simulation efforts. This makes moving through the loop slow and toilsome. What I think we need to do is to dig very deeply into basic physical and chemical phenomena to come up with new ways of interrogating biological matter in ways that productively impedance match what we are able to do in terms of IT structures and simulations. The idea is to engineer these components to work as a harmonious whole. We need to think about ways of making complex, multidimensional experiments as simple to perform as working a spreadsheet—and this is a very tough problem.

I was talking with Jeff Duyk and it turns out he has an article coming out in *Nature* where he talks about CAD/CAM—Computer-Aided Design/Computer-Aided Manufacturing. This is how CAD/CAM works. An engineer sits down at a computer terminal and in cyberspace designs an object. He defines the components of the design and analytical tools within the software to enable a suite of structural analysis tools to consider his design, or his "hypothesis." Next, the finished file is transferred to a computer controlled system that automatically creates the object, or performs the complex "experiment" for you. Basically you do not conduct the "experiment," but can directly interact with the results.

For example, a few years ago I found out about a device that rasters a laser beam, sort of like a laser printer, but instead of putting black toner onto a piece of paper it rasters over a pool photo-reactive polymer. The process repeats the rastering process on top of successive layers of un-cured liquid polymer. Eventually a complex object appears after a num-ber of layers have been completed, producing something that you can hold and play with. It was as if you had machined the object, but you did not have to be a machinist. All you had to do is sit at the computer and create that object that you could put in your pocket. I find this truly amazing.

So why don't we use these approaches to develop biological CAD/ CAM? Schematically, we can imagine the following: a scientist interac-tively runs through hypotheses by sitting at a computer system employ-ing databases and simulation tools. The next step would be for the system to guide the scientist through complex experimental designs for which the intelligent system would "assemble" and run to validate hypotheses. The experiment "assembler" is a direct interface for cyberspace to directly conceive and control experimental activities.

Let me sketch out this concept of an experiment assembler in some detail. In the 1400s, printing in Europe was done though woodblocks, a time-consuming process. In order to meet the demand for the printed page, Gutenberg developed the letterpress and the concept of movable type, avoiding the need to make a whole new plate in order to print something like a newspaper or a book. What we need in terms of our experiments is something similar to movable type, with multiple copies of very large-scale experimental motifs that you can physically move around and bring into juxtaposition. This is actually a major problem in terms of sample handling, which, when solved, would obviate significant robotic intervention. In essence, you want to develop complex experi-mental systems that intrinsically self-assemble, or are very simple to ma-nipulate in terms of bringing disparate experimental motifs, or compo-nents, together in a controllable way by the experiment assembler. (At the University of Wisconsin, we are developing components for the experi-mental assembler, in terms of systems that can either self-assemble or are simple to manipulate in terms of bringing massive numbers of experi-mental components together in a logical way.) Again, in terms of the scheme I am describing here, you would start with experimental motifs consisting of cells, peptides, nucleic acid, chemical libraries and so on. The assembler puts your experiment together, and is run creating a dense, multidimensional flux of data—this will certainly require radically new detection schemes. The data streams back into your system to validate aspects of your hypotheses, and to develop further experiments to refine this fit, or to spur new hypotheses. If we can do this, we can create many loops, and greatly accelerate the number and complexity of candidates that are truly developed in a complete biological way.

The origin of this talk stems from the fact that I am very jealous of my colleagues in the industry. I am very jealous of the fact that they have the means to pursue very large screens and to create very large datasets. I want to be able to create this in my laboratory. Industry has done a great job in development and discovery, and academia has done a great job in hypotheses development. Both sides are crossing over into the domains of the other. The activities of the Markey Scholars are a testimonial to this process.

I believe, however, that industry will always have superior resources and organization to pursue these problems and the reasons are all obviously based on economic considerations. It is a lot different writing a RO1 and getting funded, as opposed to going after a drug that can yield perhaps a billion dollars in profit.

Signal Transduction in Bacteria

Ann Stock, Ph.D.
Howard Hughes Medical Institute and
The University of Medicine and Dentistry of New Jersey
Robert Wood Johnson Medical School

TWO-COMPONENT SIGNAL TRANSDUCTION

The focus of this presentation will be signal transduction in bacteria. Signal transduction is something that we commonly associate with eukaryotic systems, but nowhere is it more important than in the prokaryotic world where single-celled organisms such as bacteria are constantly faced with dramatic changes in their environment. In order to be able to compete, survive, and thrive in their environment, they need to elicit appropriate adaptive responses to changing environmental conditions.

A majority of signal transduction in bacteria is mediated by phosphotransfer signaling systems, commonly referred to as "two-component" signal transduction pathways. These systems involve two conserved protein components. The first component is a histidine protein kinase that autophosphorylates at a histidine residue, creating a high-energy phosphoryl group that is poised for transfer to the next component. The phosphorylation of the kinase is not stoichiometric; it does not regulate the kinase activity as does phosphorylation of eukaryotic kinases. Rather, in this particular case, phosphorylation serves to provide phosphoryl groups for transfer to the second component, a protein called the response regulator.

In bacteria, these systems largely replace the small GTPase signaling pathways (such as those involving members of the ras super family) that are prevalent in eukaryotes. The response regulator functions as a phosphorylation-activated switch to control the output responses. The phosphorylated protein has a relatively short lifetime. The protein is phosphorylated at an aspartate residue, a high-energy modification that has a half-life of several hours. The chemical stability of the aspartyl phosphate is often further reduced in these systems by both intrinsic autophosphatase activity within the response regulator and by auxiliary phosphatase proteins, resulting in half-lives that range from seconds to hours in different signaling systems.

Two-component systems are very widespread throughout the bacterial kingdom. In a typical genome there are about twenty to thirty of these regulatory systems that are involved in many different functions. Some of these are housekeeping functions, but in addition, these proteins are often involved in the regulation of expression of various types of toxins and virulence factors, and in mediating antibiotic resistance through a variety of different mechanisms. This regulation is important for host-pathogen interactions.

These proteins are present and abundant in bacteria and are present to a limited extent in some eukaryotic cells. They have been found in yeasts, and in the slime mold *Dictyostelium*. They are quite prevalent in plants, but they have not been identified in animals. And this, of course, makes them promising targets for the development of antimicrobial agents.

There are a very large number of these systems that have been identified. There are well over a thousand different two-component systems that have been found in a variety of bacterial genomes; not surprisingly, like components of any signal transduction system, these proteins are incredibly modular in nature. The conserved domains can be assembled in a variety of different ways into proteins, and the proteins can be assembled in a variety of ways into pathways, creating diverse and complex schemes.

In a typical system, consisting of just two components, the histidine kinase is a transmembrane protein with a variable extracellular sensing domain and a conserved intracellular kinase domain. Phosphoryl transfer occurs to the conserved domain of the response regulator that in turn, controls the activity of an associated variable effector domain. The response regulator protein is often a transcription factor that regulates expression of a specific group of genes.

In other systems, these components can be arrayed in a much more complex fashion with multiple kinases feeding into single response regulators, single kinases feeding into multiple-response regulators, and in many cases, multiple modules allowing for multiple transfers from histidine to aspartate residues in what are known as phospho-relay schemes.

In eukaryotic two-component systems, this kind of multiple phospho-relay is the norm rather than the exception and the phospho-relay systems often interface with more conventional eukaryotic signaling pathways. For instance, in the yeast osmoregulation system, the response regulator feeds into a Map kinase cascade. In *Dictyostelium*, one response regulator contains an effector domain with phosphodiesterase activity and the two-component pathway ties into a cyclic-neucleotide signaling cascade.

The modularity of these proteins allows us to study them as individual components. The family of response regulators, with well over a thousand members to study, provides an opportunity to understand similarities and differences in the regulation of very large families. Response regulators have been the focus of research in our laboratory for a number of years, with one particular question in mind. How has nature designed a generic phosphorylation-activated switch that is capable of controlling the activity of a variety of different effector domains that are quite diverse with respect to both structure and function? Several different types of effector domains have been characterized biochemically and structurally. Examples of distinct effector domains that can be controlled by this common regulatory domain include different subfamilies of DNA-binding domains, as well as enzymes.

We know a substantial amount about the functioning of the isolated regulatory domain from research that has accumulated in a number of laboratories over quite a number of years. The domain is a simple doubly-wound beta/alpha fold. There is a cluster of highly conserved aspartic acid residues that coordinates a Mg^{2+}, creating the active site of the protein. It is this conserved response regulator domain that is actually responsible for the catalysis of phosphoryl transfer from the histidine kinase, specifically to an aspartic acid residue that is located at the C-terminal end of the third and central beta strand.

There is also another set of conserved residues that are located on adjacent beta strands 3445, creating a diagonal path leading away from the active site. These residues are a hydroxyl containing residue, either serine or threonine, and an aromatic residue, either phenylalanine or tyrosine. Over the past couple of years the roles of these conserved residues have been illuminated by structures of several isolated regulatory domains in their active states, determined in a number of different laboratories. These additional conserved residues leading from the active site function as switches that help drive a conformational change in the domain.

The conformations of these switch residues differ in inactive and active states of the domain. In the phosphorylated or activated state, the hydroxyl of the serine or threonine is positioned to form a hydrogen bond with the phosphate oxygen of the phosphorylated aspartate. The phenylalanine or tyrosine has flipped from an outward orientation to an inward orientation occupying the cavity that has been vacated by the movement of the serine or threonine. An animation demonstrates the reorientation of these residues in the active and inactive states of the regulatory domain.

A minor conformational change in the backbone accompanies the flipping of these residues. The reorientation of the residues creates a conserved mechanism for the propagation of a conformational change that, in the study of four different proteins, has been found to affect a relatively large surface, involving approximately half of the molecule. The regions showing the most change involve the 3445 surface of the domain. The backbone deviations in the region that changes conformation as a result of phosphorylation range from one to several Å, at most. The changes are relatively subtle, but they create a sufficiently distinct surface that the different surfaces can be exploited for protein-protein interactions that are specific to one state or another. This allows the regulatory domain to function as a relatively versatile switch for regulation of events that can be controlled by differential protein-protein interactions.

Our laboratory has been interested in trying to understand the details of how the altered surfaces of the regulatory domain are used for regulating different effector domain functions. A large number of structures of isolated regulatory and effector domains have been determined. There are dozens of structures of isolated regulatory domains and about a half dozen structures of isolated effector domains in the Protein Data Bank. But the structures of intact multidomain-response regulators have been relatively resistant to structural analysis. Thus the majority of what we know about the regulation of effector domain activity by regulatory domains has come from a variety of different biochemical rather than structural approaches.

Again, this family with well over a thousand members allows us an opportunity to begin to ask: "within a conserved structural family, how similar or different are the mechanisms of regulation?" If we understand how one of these proteins is regulated, does it provide an understanding of how other proteins in the same family are regulated? This is a question that is becoming increasingly important in this era of structural genomics and proteomics, where we would like to be able to extrapolate common mechanisms of function from known structural relationships.

I would like to discuss two brief stories about some of the studies that we have conducted with two representative response regulator proteins. One of them is the chemotaxis methylesterase CheB and the other, is a member of the OmpR/PhoB family of transcription factors.

REGULATION OF CHEMOTAXIS METHYLESTERASE CHEB

Before I get into the details of the methylesterase CheB, let me tell you about the system in which it functions. It belongs to the pathway of bacterial chemotaxis, which is a very extensively studied signal transduction system that is built on a two-component phosphotransfer scheme. Chemotaxis has long been advertised as a relatively simple sensory system for the study of signal transduction. However, it actually has some relatively complex regulatory features, one of which is the phenomenon of adaptation.

The receptors in the chemotaxis system signal in response to changes in ligand occupancy, not in response to absolute ligand occupancy. That is, if we follow the behavior of cells upon administering an attractant stimulus, going from a low level of stimulus up to a higher level of stimulus, we see that the cells have a steady state behavior, followed by a transient physiological response, and then adapt back to their pre-stimulus behavior. To the extent that this is occurring at the level of the receptors, this implies that receptors at a low level of occupancy and at a high level of occupancy are capable of giving the same signaling output. In this system that signaling output is the regulation of the activity of the histidine kinase. We know that this phenomenon of adaptation is facilitated by the reversible covalent modification of receptors, specifically the methylation and demethylation of specific glutamate residues within the cytoplasmic domains of the receptors.

In a very simple scheme, one can view the mechanism of adaptation in terms of a "balance model" for the receptor. In this scheme, the signaling activity of the receptor is reflective of both the ligand bound state of the receptor, and the modification state of the cytoplasmic domain. The pre-stimulus steady state is characterized by a balance between these two features. Upon addition of attractant, ligand occupancy outweighs methylation and the signaling state of the receptor is perturbed, leading to the response. Subsequently, methylation increases, counterbalancing the increased ligand and leading to a return to the pre-stimulus signaling state of the receptor. Thus adaptation is achieved, with a higher level of ligand occupancy compensated for by an increase in the level of receptor methylation. This, of course, requires that there is a very tight coupling between changes in chemo-effector level and the methylation system. So the methylation system is highly regulated.

Reversible methylation involves two enzymes: a methyltransferase and a methylesterase. The majority of the regulation is contributed by the demethylating enzyme, the methylesterase, and involves a two-component pathway. In the chemotaxis system there are actually two-response regulators that obtain phosphoryl groups from the single histidine kinase. The chemoreceptors, through a coupling protein, control the activity of the histidine kinase CheA, which passes phosphoryl groups to CheY, which acts at the flagellar motor to induce the physiological response. At the same time, phosphoryl groups are passed to the methylesterase CheB, activating it to demethylate the receptors and attenuate the response.

So how does phosphorylation work to activate the methylesterase? We know that the regulatory domain actually plays two roles in regulation of methylesterase activity. The intact unphosphorylated methylesterase has very low receptor demethylation activity. If the unphosphorylated regulatory domain is removed by genetic deletion or proteolysis, a 10-fold increase in demethylation activity is observed, indicating that the unphosphorylated regulatory domain serves as an inhibitor of the catalytic domain.

The demethylation activity of the phosphorylated intact protein is tenfold greater than that of the isolated catalytic domain. The phosphorylated domain enhances the activity of the catalytic domain. So there are actually two roles for the regulatory domain: an inhibitory activity of the unphosphorylated domain, and an activating function of the phosphorylated domain.

The crystal structure of CheB, determined by postdoctoral fellows Senzana Djorjdevic and Ann West, has provided insight to the basis of the inhibitory interaction. A space-filling model of structure of the intact methylesterase illustrates a very tight packing of the regulatory domain against the catalytic domain, almost completely blocking access to the catalytic triad of the active site. In a modeling experiment, we attempted to dock the methylation region of the receptor, specifically a helix with glutamate residues, near the active site serine nucleophile of the catalytic domain. However, the glutamate residues cannot approach closer than ~7 Å without steric collision.

The interface between the regulatory and catalytic domains is a tightly packed interface that has extensive contacts, hydrophobic in the center and more hydrophilic at the periphery. Notably, the core of the domain interface is formed by a pair of phenylalanine residues. The phenylalanine contributed by the regulatory domain is the conserved aromatic residue that in phosphorylated response regulators is part of the switch mechanism, flipping from an outward orientation in the inactive state to an inward orientation in the phosphorylated state. We anticipate that reorientation of this residue would disrupt the domain interface, exposing the active site for interaction with the receptor substrate.

We wanted to probe this mechanism of activation. However, the short lifetime of the phosphorylated state of this protein, with a half-life of only one second, makes it relatively difficult to approach the structure of the phosphorylated state by conventional means. So Ganesh Anand, a graduate student in my laboratory, collaborated with Betsy Komives at UCSD to use a method of deuterium exchange analyzed by mass spectrometry to characterize solvent accessibility at the domain interface upon phosphorylation.

In these deuterium exchange experiments, the protein is quenched at low pH, digested with pepsin, and then peptic fragments are isolated and analyzed by mass spectrometry. If the protein is briefly incubated in the presence of deuterium before this analysis, deuterons are exchanged for protons at solvent accessible backbone amides. The deuterium-substituted peptides, indicative of regions of increased solvent exposure, are shifted to higher masses relative to their hydrogen-containing counterparts. Various times of incubation in deuterium can be employed to generate rates of deuterium incorporation into different peptides.

This analysis was performed on the methylesterase CheB in the absence of phosphorylation and under conditions of steady-state phosphorylation. As is typical of this method, there were a small number of peptides for which no quantitative data could be determined, but we obtained fairly complete coverage. The majority of the peptides showed no changes in deuterium-exchange rates upon phosphorylation. Two peptides showed increased solvent exchange upon phosphorylation. Both were located within the catalytic domain at the interdomain interface. When mapped onto the surface of the catalytic domain, it is apparent that these peptides form two edges of the domain interface. These regions become more solvent exposed upon phosphorylation, but not nearly as solvent exposed as what we observed in the isolated catalytic domain.

These data indicate that the domains do readjust their orientation in the phosphorylated state. However, they do not separate completely. There is a substantial interface that remains between the two domains, perhaps providing a path for allosteric communication between the regulatory domain and the active site of the catalytic domain. Such contact may mediate the 10-fold activation contributed by the phosphorylated domain.

THE OMPR/PHOB FAMILY OF TRANSCRIPTION FACTORS

The chemotaxis system is a somewhat atypical two-component system. The two response regulators of the chemotaxis system are unusual in that they are not transcription factors. The vast majority of response regulators in two-component systems are responsible for regulation of gene expression and the effector domains of these response regulators are DNA-binding domains. The bacterial response regulators can be divided into subfamilies based on homology within their C-terminal DNA-binding domains.

A survey of the *E. coli* genome conducted by Mizuno several years ago, revealed that out of the 32 response regulators in *E. coli*, 25 of them could be categorized as belonging to the previously identified three subfamilies of transcription factors based on homology within their DNA-binding domains. One of these three families, the OmpR/PhoB family, accounts for approximately 40 percent of all response regulators in bacterial genomes. This subfamily is characterized by a DNA-binding domain with a winged-helix fold. The OmpR/PhoB group is by far the largest subfamily. There are two other smaller subfamilies of transcription factors with different types of DNA-binding domains. A small number of proteins are unrelated to other response regulators and are grouped into a miscellaneous category. The two chemotaxis proteins discussed above are members of this group.

We are interested in the large family of transcription factors represented by the OmpR/PhoB subfamily. The family is named after the OmpR protein that participates in osmoregulation in *E. coli*. The osmoregulation system involves a histidine kinase EnvZ that is a transmembrane kinase that senses changes in osmotic strength. EnvZ provides phosphoryl groups to the response regulator OmpR, which functions as a transcription factor. The C-terminal, or effector, domain of this response regulator is a DNA-binding domain, and OmpR, in its phosphorylated state, binds in a hierarchical fashion to binding sites that are located upstream of the genes that encode the major outer membrane porin proteins, OmpF and OmpC. These proteins are regulated not in a single on-off switch fashion, but in a much more subtle way. At low osmotic strength, there is a high level of expression of *ompF*. At high-osmotic strength, there is a high level of expression of *ompC*. Expression of these genes is differentially coordinated so that the total concentration of porin proteins remains constant while the composition varies.

The OmpR protein serves as both an activator and repressor of transcription, depending on the binding sites that are occupied. Each of the binding sites preceding the *ompF* and *ompC* genes consists of two ten-base pair half-sites arranged as direct repeats.

Structural analysis of the DNA-binding domain of OmpR by Erik Martínez-Hackert, a graduate student in my laboratory, defined the winged-helix fold for this family. Several experiments including site-specific cleavage analysis allowed us to predict a model for the interaction of this DNA-binding domain with its recognition sites in DNA. This model, though useful, is incomplete. In the cell, the phosphorylated regulatory domain is required for efficient DNA binding and transcriptional regulation. We would like to understand the specific role of the regulatory domain in allowing the DNA-binding domain to interact with its DNA sites.

Despite the fact that this is a huge family of transcription factors with over 500 members, and a number of laboratories have been pursuing structures of different family members, these proteins have been quite resistant to crystallization. David Buckler, a postdoctoral fellow in my laboratory, finally made progress in this pursuit by using proteins from the thermophilic bacterium, *Thermotoga maritima*. When the *Thermotoga* genome was reported, it was possible to clone all of the response regulator members that belonged to the OmpR/PhoB family. There are four of these proteins. David expressed and purified all of them, and was lucky enough to be able to crystallize one. The structure of this protein, DrrD, revealed no particular surprises with regard to the folds of the individual domains.

What was of interest was the orientation of the regulatory domain with respect to the DNA-binding domain. In this regard, the structure was surprising. In the crystal structure, the regulatory domain packs against the DNA-binding domain via an extremely small interface. There are only 250 Å^2 of buried surface area. This value falls substantially below the area of any bona fide domain interface observed in any monomeric protein in the Protein Data Bank. The interface in DrrD is much smaller than the typical size of a domain interface, which would be ~1200 Å^2.

Of course, in a crystal structure, there needs to be an interaction between domains. Proteins have to be able to pack within the crystal lattice. We believe that crystallization has trapped these two domains in a fixed orientation that is not reflective of how they would exist in solution. The lack of a unique conformation would help explain why this particular OmpR/PhoB subfamily of response regulators has been so resistant to crystallization. Notably, within the very short linker that connects the two domains of DrrD together, there are two missing residues that lack electron density and the surrounding residues in the linker region have very high temperature factors. Again, these data suggest that this domain interface is not a stable interface, and that the linker that tethers the two domains to each other is flexible.

The lack of a substantial domain interface makes DrrD unique among the three response regulators that have been crystallized as intact proteins to date. Comparing the buried surface areas at the domain interfaces of these three response regulators, two have substantial interfaces of ~1000 Å^2. One of these is the chemotaxis methylesterase CheB, discussed above. The other is NarL, a transcription factor belonging to a completely different subfamily of response regulators. The structure of NarL, determined by Dick Dickerson's group, reveals an extensive domain interface. These large interfaces in these two structures contrast with the very tiny patch of buried surface between the two domains of DrrD, implying that these proteins utilize different types of regulatory interactions.

The two response regulators for which structures have been known for several years have served as a model for understanding interdomain regulation. In both cases, there are large domain interfaces and the regulatory domains pack against the C-terminal effector domains, essentially precluding access to the functional regions of the effector domains: the active site of the methylesterase CheB, and the recognition helix of the transcription factor NarL. In contrast, in DrrD, the transcription factor of the OmpR/PhoB subfamily, the recognition helix is completely unobstructed by the regulatory domain.

The structure of DrrD suggests a model for regulation that is fundamentally different than that observed for other response regulators. Rather than a mechanism of regulation involving intra-molecular communication between the regulatory and effector domains within a monomer, the regulation within DrrD, and perhaps other members of the OmpR/PhoB subfamily, appears to occur through inter-molecular interactions. Specifically, activation is proposed to proceed primarily through dimerization of the phosphorylated regulatory domains with the effector domains participating as passive partners.

Chimeric response regulators within the OmpR/PhoB subfamily, involving the regulatory domain of one member attached to the effector domain of another, have been constructed and function well, providing further support for this type of mechanism. These experiments have been performed with a limited number of OmpR/PhoB subfamily members at this point. One of the questions that remains at this time is whether within the subfamily, all members will function by a similar regulatory mechanism or whether within this large family, different members will have different mechanisms of regulation.

This study has indicated that within large structural families, although sequence and structural similarity exist, there may be some very significant differences in the way proteins function and in particular, in the specific protein-protein interaction mechanisms that are being used for regulation in signal transduction proteins.

ACKNOWLEDGMENTS

The people associated with studies of methylesterase CheB were Ganesh Anand, a graduate student who performed the biochemical analyses; and Ann West and Snezana Djordjevic, postdoctoral fellows who determined the structure. The deuterium exchange study was done in collaboration with Betsy Komives at UCSD. The people associated with analyses of the OmpR family transcription factors were Erik Martínez-Hackert and Patricia Harrison-McMonagle, graduate students who determined the structure of the DNA-binding domain and performed the cleavage analysis that allowed us to model the interaction with DNA; and David Buckler, a postdoctoral fellow who determined the structure of the intact OmpR family member, DrrD. Financial support was provided by the NIH and HHMI.

AAKI, a Novel Kinase that Regulates Cargo Selection for Clatherin-Mediated Endocytosis

Sandra Louise Schmid, Ph.D.
The Scripps Research Institute

My lab has been interested, since its beginnings, in trying to understand the process of receptor-mediated endocytosis. It involves high-affinity binding of macromolecules, like LDL receptors or even virus particles, to specific receptors on the cell surface. These receptors contain sorting motifs, different flavors of sorting motifs, as you will see later in the talk, which are recognized by coat proteins, that form the basis for an endocytic machinery. The coat proteins assemble into a polygonal lattice, which forms curved structures that help to deform and invaginate the membrane forming coated pits. Finally, membrane fission, which is regulated by the GTPase dynamin that assembles into a collar-like structure encircling the neck of deeply invaginated coated pits, releases a transport vesicle that carries concentrated cargo receptor and ligand complexes into the cell.

The major coat proteins have been identified for some time now. They are clathrin triskelions and adapter protein-2 complexes (AP2s). You can think of clathrin as the "brauns" of this machinery. It self-assembles into a polygonal lattice and by so doing drives the membrane invagination. The AP2s are the "brains" of the machinery. They recognize cargo molecules, and trigger clathrin assembly thereby coordinating vesicle formation and cargo recruitment.

In order to study how coat assembly is regulated in the cell and to identify what other factors might be involved in mediating this process of receptor-mediated endocytosis, I began, as a postdoctoral fellow with the support of the Markey Fellowship, to develop new cell free assays, using perforated A431 cells that faithfully reconstitute these events.

We have also developed stage specific biochemical assays that allow us to detect sequential intermediates in endocytic-coated vesicle formation. These assays follow the receptor-mediated endocytosis of transferrin, which is biotinylated with a cleavable disulfide bond (referred to as BSSTfn). The "sequestration" of receptor-bound BSSTfn into an intermediate in vesicle formation, called a constricted coated pit, can be detected when the ligand becomes inaccessible to avidin. However, because constricted coated pits remain accessible to small molecules through a narrow opening at their necks that connects them to the plasma membrane, the BSSTfn sequestered in them can be cleaved by the small membrane-impermeant, reducing agent, MesNa. Thus, late events in vesicle formation, namely the release of a sealed vesicle from the plasma membrane are detected when the BSSTfn becomes resistant to MesNa. Finally, we can focus on measuring the earliest events in vesicle formation, by supplementing assays performed in the presence of limiting concentrations of cytosol with purified coat proteins. The coat protein-stimulated sequestration of BSSTfn into constricted coated pits reflects de novo coat assembly.

Many years of work helped us to biochemically characterize these stages of vesicle formation. We found that while the coat proteins, clathrin and AP2, are necessary for coated vesicle formation, they are not sufficient. For example, intermediate and late events in this process are regulated by the GTPase dynamin. Most of my work in the past 6 years has focused on understanding the function in vivo and in vitro of this GTPase, although it is not subject of the talk today. These late events also require ATP hydrolysis, by an as-yet-unidentified ATPase, as well as numerous accessory proteins that have been implicated by virtue of their interaction with dynamin and with the coat proteins.

Early events in CCV formation require the lipid, phosphatidylinositol-4,5 -bisphosphate (PI-4,5-P_2), which provides at least part of the targeting signal for recruitment of AP2 complexes and other endocytic accessory proteins, including dynamin to the plasma membrane. Early events also require ATP hydrolysis and again, we have not identified the ATPase. One candidate, however, will be the subject of my talk today. The role of numerous accessory proteins that interact with adapters and clathrin are not known.

I will focus on the regulation of endocytic vesicle formation. An extremely talented postdoc, Sean Conner, did all of the work I am going to tell you about today. Because the adaptors are a key factor in initiating coat assembly—"the brains of the operation"—we focused our attention on these. The AP2 complex consists of four subunits, called alpha, beta, sigma, and mu adaptins. The alpha adaptin is involved in targeting to the plasma membrane, through interactions with both proteins and PI-4,5-P_2. The beta adaptin, particularly the hinge region, binds and triggers clathrin assembly. The N-terminal appendage domains of both the alpha and beta adaptins (also called "ear" domains as the AP2 complex looks like a Mickey mouse head with 2 alpha and beta appendage domain "ears") also bind a number of accessory molecules whose exact function in endocytosis has yet to be established. The mu subunit recognizes specific sorting motifs on cargo molecules, and in particular has been shown to recognize tyrosine-based sorting motifs such as those found in the transferrin receptor.

To identify new factors that might regulate AP2 complex function we decided to "go fishing" using the appendage domain of the alpha adaptin fused to GST as "bait." We chose the phage-display approach and cast our immobilized GST-alpha ear "fishing pole" into a phage pool. This approach allowed us to control the quality of our bait and the biochemical conditions in which we measure the interaction. Through multiple rounds of binding, elution and phage amplification we could increase the signal:noise ratio to identify specific interactions and identify less abundant molecules. All of the proteins known to interact with clathrin adaptors are very abundant-scaffolding proteins, identified from cell lysates through protein pull-down approaches. As we were interested in regulatory molecules, we took this approach to look for proteins that might be less abundant.

In addition to all the known interacting proteins, we found that 30 percent of the clones in our selected phage samples encoded a C-terminal fragment from a novel member of the serine/threonine kinase family. This multidomain protein encodes an N-terminal serine/threonine kinase domain, a central glutamine, proline and alanine-rich domain, and the C-terminal, alpha interacting domain (AID). The AID has several DPF and NPF motifs that are known to bind to the alpha ear.

We were able to verify these protein interactions in vitro showing that the C-terminal region of what we now call adapter-associated kinase one or AAK1 indeed interacts directly with the alpha appendage domain. We expressed the intact AAK1 using the baculovirus expression system and confirmed that it, like the AID alone, is able to pull down the alpha adapter from rat brain cytosol. We also made antibodies to AAK1 and showed that the protein copurifies with clathrin-coated vesicles from bovine brain and from rat liver. AAK1, together with the coat proteins, can be extracted from the membrane by Tris-buffer. When the extracted coat proteins are subsequently purified by gel filtration, we find that AAK1 copurifies with APs and not with clathrin. These studies provided the functional basis for the name, AAK1.

Immunolocalization studies in neurons established that AAK1 is enriched at sites of endocytosis, which are identified by the uptake of rhodamine-labelled dextran into activated hippocampal neurons. AAK1 colocalizes with these endocytic hot spots together with AP2 and dynamin. Endogenous AAK1 also colocalizes with the AP2 adapters on the plasma membrane in non-neuronal cells.

Based on these results, we felt very comfortable that the kinase we had identified was relevant to the process of endocytosis. What, then, is the function of AAK1? We first approached this question by asking, what are its substrates? We found in *in vitro* assays that although AAK1 binds the alpha adaptin, it specifically phosphorylates the mu subunit of the AP2 complex. In collaboration with Stefan Höning and Doris Ricotta (University of Göttingen, Germany) we identified threonine 156 as the AAK1 phosphorylation site on the mu subunit. A former postdoc of mine, Elizabeth Smythe, now leading her own lab in Shefield, had recently shown that phosphorylation of threonine 156 on the mu subunit was essential for endocytosis both in vivo and in vitro (Olusanya, O. et al. 2001. *Curr Biol.* 11:896-900), providing further evidence that AAK1 was indeed a functionally relevant kinase for endocytosis.

What are the consequences of this phosphorylation of mu? As I mentioned, the mu subunit recognizes cargo-sorting motifs on cargo molecules. Our collaborators, Doris and Stefan, therefore, looked at the affinity of AP2s for these sorting motif-containing peptides, using a BiaCore to measure surface plasmon resonance. AP2 complexes, isolated from bovine brain extracts, bind peptides containing these tyrosine-based sorting motifs with a certain affinity (116 nM). If the AP2s, which copurify with an endogenous kinase, are first treated with a phosphatase, then the binding affinity is decreased approximately five-fold. Conversely, if we incubate this preparation with ATP and allow the endogenous kinase to phophorylate mu, we see an approximate two-fold increase in binding affinity. Strikingly, incubation with purified AAK1 and ATP enhances the binding affinity of AP2 for tyrosine motif-containing peptides by 25-fold compared to phosphatase treated AP2s. From this we conclude that AAK1 phosphorylates mu on Thr156 to regulate its affinity for cargo molecules containing tyrosine-based sorting motifs.

To examine the effects of AAK1 on endocytic coated vesicle formation, we took advantage of our perforated cell system and our ability to selectively measure early events in coated-vesicle formation. In an assay in which we supplement incubations performed under limiting concentrations of cytosol with purified AP2s, adding increasing concentrations of AP2 leads to increased sequestration of BSSTfn into constricted coated pits—a measure of early events in endocytosis. When these reactions are supplemented with AAK1, the AP2-stimulated early events are significantly inhibited. If we first inactivate the AAK1 by treating it with an irreversible kinase inhibitor, FSBA, it becomes a much less potent inhibitor of the AP2-stimulated signal. Thus, excess AAK1 appears to inhibit the sequestration of receptor-bound BSSTfn into newly formed constricted coated pits.

I had previously described the work of Liz Smythe who had shown that phosphorylation of mu was necessary for endocytosis. This might seem paradoxical with our finding that adding excess AAK1 inhibits endocytosis. I will try to resolve this paradox with a model at the end of my talk. First, however, we wanted to see whether there were any other substrates that we could detect in these more complex cell extracts. When AAK1 is incubated with either cell membranes or cytosol, the principal product, other than autophosphorylation of AAK1, is the mu subunit. Thus, although we cannot rule out that there are other substrates involved, we believe that the effects on endocytosis are due primarily to the phosphorylation of mu.

Given the apparent paradox of needing AAK1-mediated phosphorylation of mu for early events in endocytosis in a perforated system, yet finding that excess active AAK1 inhibits endocytosis, we decided to look in vivo to see what the effects of AAK1 overexpression might be. To this end we constructed adenovirus expressing wild-type and mutant AAK1 kinases under the control of a tetracycline regulatable promoter so that we could control levels of expression. When either the wild type or kinase-inactive AAK1 were overexpressed using this adenoviral system, Tfn-receptor-mediated endocytosis was inhibited. The kinase-dead mutant was a less potent inhibitor than the WT AAK1, thus these *in vivo* data closely matched the results we saw in our in vitro, perforated cell system. Inhibition was not due to sequestration of some binding partner of AAK1, or to rampant kinase activity, because when we overexpressed truncation products of AAK1 lacking the AID or the AID alone, these constructs do not inhibit Tfn endocytosis.

Further characterization revealed that overexpressing either the wild-type or kinase-inactive AAK1 mutants, displaced AP2s from the coated pits. Instead of the normal punctate distribution of AP2 in coated pits, as detected by immunolocalization, the AP2 staining becomes diffuse. Subcellular fractionation studies established that although the AP2 complexes were no longer clustered into coated pits, they remained associated with the plasma membrane and the relative distribution between the membrane pool and the cytosolic pool was unchanged by overexpressing either the wild-type or mutant kinase.

Surprisingly, while AP2 distribution in coated pits was disrupted, the distribution of clathrin was not affected. This finding goes against that expected by the dogma that AP2s are responsible for triggering clathrin assembly. In cells overexpressing AAK1, clathrin appears to assemble in the absence of AP2 clustering. But are these coated pits still functional?

The mu subunit recognizes tyrosine-based sorting motifs and phosphorylation by AAK1 enhances the affinity for those sorting motifs 25-fold, therefore we decided to look at another cargo molecule, which has a different kind of sorting motif. Endocytosis of EGF receptors is known to occur through clathrin-coated pits. Indeed, double label immunoelectron microscopy shows that EGF receptors are found in the same coated pits as transferrin receptors. However, in contrast to the Tfn receptor, endocytosis of EGF receptors is ligand dependent and not affected by mutations in mu that disrupt their ability to bind tyrosine-based sorting motifs. We therefore looked at EGF uptake and found that it was unaffected by AAK1 overexpression. As a positive control, we overexpressed a dominant negative dynamin mutant that potently inhibits both EGF and Tfn receptor uptake. These findings were confirmed microscopically using fluorescently-labeled EGF or Tfn as endocytic tracers, in which cells overexpressing AAK1 fail to efficiently take up fluorescent-Tfn molecules, but continue to take up fluoresent-EGF molecules. Together these data suggest that AAK1 can selectively regulate clathrin-mediated endocytosis of different cargo molecules.

We heard from Dan Madison yesterday another striking example of cargo selective regulation of endocytosis as he described the regulation of postsynaptic NMDA receptor endocytic trafficking by calcium-dependent phosphatases and kinases that function to control the levels of AMPA receptor expression and responses to neurotransmitters.

Thus, a new concept emerging from these studies is the existence of cargo-selected regulation of uptake into the cell. The AAK1 kinase is one of the first mechanistically described examples of this regulation. Importantly, AAK1 appears to regulate endocytosis of transferrin receptors, which are nutrient receptors classically defined as being constitutively endocytosed. Thus, the "constitutive" endocytic pathway is, in fact, subject to regulation.

Our current working model to explain all of the observations we have, not all of which I have described to you, is that the effective concentration of cargo molecules into coated pits requires cycles of phosphorylation and dephosphorylation of the mu subunit, mediated by AAK1. The recently published three-dimensional structure of the AP2 core (Collins, B.M., et al. 2002. *Cell* 109:523-35) suggests a mechanism by which phosphorylation at Thr156 in a linker region of mu subunit induces a conformational change to expose the otherwise buried tyrosine-motif binding site in the molecule. In this way, phosphorylation is thought to be required for high-affinity binding to cargo molecules at the surface. Once bound to cargo molecules, subsequent dephosphorylation of AP2 complexes may be required to allow the AP2s to self-associate and/or to trigger clathrin assembly and vesicle formation.

We propose then that the kinase inactive mutant blocks cargo recruitment at an early stage in coated vesicle formation, and that overexpression of wildtype AAK1 blocks at a subsequent step. Our future efforts will be directed towards testing this model and elucidating the role of AAK1 in regulating clathrin-mediated endocytosis.

NOTE: The following papers report some of the studies described here, Conner, S. D., and S. L. Schmid. 2002. *J Cell Biol.* 156:921-9; and Ricotta, D. et al. 2002. *J Cell Biol.* 156:791-5. Conner, S. D. and S. L. Schmid. 2003. *J Cell Biol.* 162:773-80.

Abstracts of
Poster Sessions

CONFIGURATIONAL ENTROPY, BIOCHEMICAL COOPERATIVITY, AND SIGNAL TRANSDUCTION

Paul H. Axelsen, M.D.
Department of Pharmacology
University of Pennsylvania

Cooperativity is a common biochemical phenomenon in which two or more otherwise independent processes are thermodynamically coupled. Because cooperative processes are usually attended by changes in molecular conformation, thermodynamic coupling is usually attributed to an enthalpy-driven mechanism. In the family of glycopeptide antibiotics that includes vancomycin, however, cooperative phenomena occur that cannot be explained by conformational change. We have demonstrated that cooperativity in these systems can arise solely from changes in vibrational activity using molecular dynamics simulation. This result has important implications for much larger systems because ligand-induced modulation of periodic motions in a macromolecular system is an eminently plausible means of communicating the presence of bound ligand over long distances. Indeed, the function of large membrane proteins such as those involved in transmembrane signal transduction may actually require a mechanism based on configurational entropy changes because the enthalpy changes generally involved in the binding of small ligands are small compared to the magnitude of potential energy fluctuations one would expect in systems of this size.

EMBRYONIC BEGINNINGS OF THE HEMATOPOIETIC AND VASCULAR SYSTEMS DURING MOUSE DEVELOPMENT

Margaret H. Baron, M.D., Ph.D.
Department of Medicine, Biochemistry and Molecular Biology
Mount Sinai School of Medicine

Blood and vascular endothelial cells form in all vertebrates during gastrulation, a process in which the mesoderm of the embryo is induced and then patterned by molecules whose identity is still largely unknown. "Blood islands" of primitive hematopoietic cell clusters surrounded by a layer of endothelial cells form in the yolk sac, external to the developing embryo proper (epiblast). These lineages arise from a layer of extra embryonic mesoderm that is closely apposed with a layer of primitive (visceral) endoderm. Despite the identification of genes such as *Flk1, SCL/tal-*

1, *Cbfa2/Runx1/AML1* and *CD34* that are expressed during the induction of primitive hematopoiesis and vasculogenesis, the early molecular and cellular events involved in these processes are not well understood. We demonstrated previously that specification of these lineages requires a signal(s) secreted from the adjacent visceral endoderm (VE) and more recently that Indian hedgehog (Ihh) is a VE-secreted signal which alone is sufficient to induce formation of hematopoietic and endothelial cells. We have continued to investigate the mechanism by which Ihh activates these processes. As seen with VE, Ihh can also respecify prospective neural ectoderm (anterior epiblast) along hematopoietic and endothelial (posterior) lineages, as indicated by cell morphology, activation of specific transgenes (e.g., *lacZ* reporters controlled by embryonic *globin*, *Flk1* and *Cbfa2/Runx1/AML1* sequences), activation of endogenous markers of stem/progenitor cells (hemangioblasts) and more differentiated cells, and by immunostaining for PECAM1 and other proteins. Dispersed cells from recombinant human IHH-treated anterior epiblasts form primitive or definitive hematopoietic colonies in secondary cultures in the presence of appropriate cytokines, indicating that functional hematopoietic stem cells are produced, and endothelial cell sprouting is observed. As expected, downstream targets of the Hh signaling pathway (*Ptch1, Smo, Gli1*) are upregulated in anterior epiblasts cultured in the presence of Ihh protein. Blocking Ihh function in VE inhibits activation of hematopoiesis and vasculogenesis in the adjacent epiblast, suggesting that Ihh is an endogenous signal that plays a key role in the development of the earliest hemato-vascular system. The gene encoding Bone morphogenetic protein-4 (Bmp-4) is upregulated in the target epiblast in response to Ihh. Several more direct lines of evidence indicate that Ihh functions, at least in part, through activation of the Bmp signaling pathway. *Hedgehog* genes and protein are expressed by adult mouse and human bone marrow stromal cells and *Ptch1* and *Smo* are expressed in hematopoietic stem/progenitor as well as endothelial cells. Therefore, these findings may have important implications for regulating hematopoiesis and vascular development for practical and therapeutic purposes.

FLUORESCENCE DETECTION TECHNOLOGIES AND BIOMEDICAL RESEARCH: PROTEOMICS, GENOMICS, IMAGING, ARRAYS, AND DISEASE

Joseph M. Beechem, Ph.D.
Molecular Probes, Inc.

In 1981, when I started graduate school at The Johns Hopkins University (Baltimore, MD), fluorescence spectroscopy was a technique mainly practiced by biophysicists. Everyone else in my graduate school class was "flocking-to" laboratories in really hot-areas of research, which at that time was molecular biology/genetics. During my Ph.D. training, instead of learning the latest cloning technique or expression system, items such as: fluorescence polarization/anisotropy, fluorescence resonance energy-transfer (FRET), excited-state reactions, solvent relaxation, protein folding, fast kinetics, etc., formed the heart of my research. The relevance of these "arcane" spectroscopic methodologies for biomedical research was tenuous (at best). Fortunately, as modern biomedical research methodologies evolved, these "arcane" fluorescence spectroscopic techniques became some of the key detection technologies associated with much of the modern biomedical research "revolution." Fluorescence polarization /anisotropy spectroscopy has become an essential component of high throughput homogenous drug screening and protein-protein interaction assays. Fluorescence energy-transfer (FRET) became the key technology behind molecular "beacons," and high-sensitivity DNA microarray techniques. Ultra-high sensitivity protein folding dyes are becoming the core technology associated with proteomics platform imaging of 2-D gels. Fluorophores covalently coupled to chelating reagents formed the key technology associated with discovering the important role of calcium as a universal "currency" of intracellular signaling. The list goes on-and-on and, most importantly, many key applications of fluorescence technology to biomedical research *have yet to be developed*. In this presentation, data will be described for the "next generation" of fluorescence reagents and methodologies, which are being developed at Molecular Probes. From high resolution deconvolved intracellular imaging of organelles, to mass-spectroscopy/fluorescence-combined approaches for whole cell post-translational modification mapping will be presented. These (and additional) fluorescence technologies will continue to play an active role in helping biomedical research solve the major health problems facing the modern world.

IDENTIFICATION OF THE PROTEIN 4.2 GENE AS A DIRECT TARGET OF THE TAL1/CL TRANSCRIPTION FACTOR IN DIFFERENTIATING MURINE ERYTHROID CELLS

Zhixiong Xu and Stephen J. Brandt, M.D.
Vanderbilt University and Veterans Affairs Medical Centers

The *TAL1/SCL* gene, originally identified through its involvement by a recurrent chromosomal translocation in leukemic T-cells, encodes a basic helix-loop-helix (bHLH) transcription factor essential for embryonic hematopoiesis and vascular remodeling. Although TAL1 is presumed to alter the transcription of a specific set of genes, no such targets have been definitively identified. Binding site selection assays using erythroid cell extracts have suggested that TAL1 contributes to a multi-protein DNA-binding complex that binds preferentially to a tandem E box (for bHLH proteins)-GATA motif and which also contains the zinc finger transcription factor GATA-1, the LIM domain protein LMO2, and the LIM domain binding protein Ldb1. We identified two such E box-GATA elements in the proximal promoter of the murine Protein 4.2 gene whose protein product plays an important role in maintaining the stability and flexibility of erythrocytes. To determine if transcription of this gene is regulated by such a complex, we analyzed the contributions of TAL1 and GATA-1 to Protein 4.2 DNA binding activity, promoter activity, and endogenous gene expression and *in vivo* occupancy of the Protein 4.2 promoter by TAL1. First, several TAL1-, GATA1-, LMO2-, and Ldb1-containing complexes were detected by gel mobility shift analysis of erythroid cell extracts using probes corresponding to either E box-GATA element in the Protein 4.2 promoter. An increase in these DNA-binding activities was observed with DMSO-induced differentiation of murine erythroleukemia (MEL) cells concomitant with expression of Protein 4.2 mRNA. Cold competitor studies and gel mobility shift assays with mutant probes indicated a requirement for both the E box and GATA sites in formation of these binding complexes and revealed an increased stability for the ternary complex relative to other E box- and GATA-binding complexes in MEL nuclear extracts. Using a novel modification of the gel mobility shift assay, it was shown that this TAL1- and GATA-containing complex could bridge in solution two double-stranded oligonucleotide probes corresponding to the two E box-GATA elements in the Protein 4.2 promoter. Reporter gene assays showed that DMSO-induced promoter activity was decreased by 75 percent and 90 percent, respectively, with mutation of either E box or GATA site, suggesting that both E box-GATA elements contribute to promoter activity and that both the E box and GATA sites within these elements are required for maximal induction of Protein 4.2

gene expression during MEL cell differentiation. In addition, a TAL1 expression vector increased Protein 4.2 promoter activity when cotransfected with vectors for its DNA-binding partner E47, GATA-1, LMO2, and Ldb1. Finally, an increase in endogenous Protein 4.2 gene expression and in E box-GATA DNA-binding activities was observed when TAL1 was overexpressed in MEL cells, a decrease in both was observed with enforced expression of a TAL1 mutant defective in DNA-binding or an Ldb1 mutant impaired in dimerization, and evidence for *in vivo* occupancy of the Protein 4.2 promoter by TAL1 was obtained through chromatin immunoprecipitation analysis. In sum, these data establish the Protein 4.2 gene as a direct target of a TAL1- and GATA-1-containing DNA-binding complex in differentiating erythroid cells.

CELL SIGNALING NETWORKS IN
C. ELEGANS MORPHOGENESIS

Andrew Chisholm, Ph.D., Ian Chin-Sang, Mei Ding, Sean George,
Bob Harrington, Tom Holcomb, Kris Larsen, and Sarah Moseley
Department of Biology
University of California

The epidermis of the nematode *C. elegans* is a simple model for analyzing mechanisms of epithelial morphogenesis. The worm epidermis undergoes several distinct morphogenetic movements, including epiboly, cell intercalation, directed dilation, and invagination. We have focused on the epiboly movements required for epidermal enclosure of the embryo. The epidermis develops from a sheet of cells lying on the dorsal part of the embryo. Changes in epidermal cell shape cause the epidermis to expand laterally and ventrally, moving over neuronal substrate cells. This results in epidermal enclosure in the embryo at the ventral midline. Using genetics we have found that signaling between underlying neuronal precursors is important for normal enclosure.

Mutations in the *C. elegans* Eph receptor VAB-1 and the ephrin ligand VAB-2/EFN-1 cause defects in neural and epidermal morphogenesis (George et al., 1998 *Cell* 92:633; Chin-Sang, et al., 1999 *Cell* 99:781). VAB-1 and VAB-2 are expressed in complementary sets of neurons during embryogenesis, and are required in neurons for epidermal morphogenesis. VAB-1 may have kinase-dependent and kinase-independent functions; *vab-2* mutations synergise with *vab-1* kinase domain mutations and not with a *vab-1* extracellular domain mutation, suggesting that VAB-2 may mediate a kinase-independent function of VAB-1.

The almost complete *C. elegans* genome encodes one Eph receptor (VAB-1) and four GPI-anchored ephrins (EFN-1/VAB-2, EFN-2, EFN-3, and EFN-4). Mutations in the gene *mab-26* cause morphogenetic defects related to but distinct from those seen in *vab-1* and *vab-2* mutants. We have shown that *mab-26* corresponds to the fourth worm ephrin (EFN-4). Strikingly, *mab-26* mutations display synthetic lethality with *vab-1* and *vab-2* mutations, suggesting that MAB-26 may function in VAB-1-independent signaling.

Loss of function in the *C. elegans* LAR-like receptor tyrosine phosphatase PTP-1 causes morphogenetic defects. We have found that *ptp-1* mutants display synthetic lethality with *vab-1, vab-2,* and *mab-26* mutations. These results suggest that RPTP signaling may function in a parallel redundant pathway with Eph signaling. We are currently testing whether this interaction is specific to the Eph signaling mutants.

PAS PROTEINS AND THE REGULATION OF DEVELOPMENT AND PHYSIOLOGY

Stephen Crews, Ph.D.
Department of Biochemistry and Biophysics
University of North Carolina, Chapel Hill

The central nervous system consists of a large variety of neuronal and glial cell types. Neural precursor cells are first specified and those precursors then generate distinct CNS cell types. We have studied the formation of the cells that lie along the midline of the *Drosophila* CNS. This work has lead to an understanding of how distinct regions of the CNS are generated and the discovery of a class of regulatory proteins that control a wide variety of invertebrate and vertebrate developmental and physiological processes.

Single-minded and the control of CNS midline cell development. The CNS midline cells comprise a distinct set of functional neurons and glia, and also act as a signaling center that controls aspects of axon guidance, cell migration, and formation of epidermal, mesodermal, and neural cell types. We have broadly investigated CNS midline cell development using genetics and molecular techniques to identify and functionally analyze genes involved in establishing midline cell fate and function. The *single-minded* gene acts as a master regulator of CNS midline cell transcription and formation. Dorsal/ventral patterning proteins act in a concentration-dependent and cooperative mode in conjunction with the *Notch* signaling pathway to activate *single-minded* transcription in midline precursor cells.

The *single-minded* gene encodes a basic-helix-loop-helix-PAS transcription factor that is required for all transcription and development of the midline cells. Single-minded protein dimerizes with the Tango bHLH-PAS protein. Together they enter the nucleus, bind to DNA control elements containing an ACGTG core sequence, and activate midline transcription in conjunction with additional unknown coregulators. Correct formation of the CNS midline cells involves activation of midline gene transcription and repression of lateral CNS transcription in the midline cells. Single-minded is required for both processes: it activates transcription of midline-expressed genes and the transcription of repressive factors. Single-minded continues to function throughout development. As midline precursor cells differentiate, the Single-minded: Tango protein complex interacts combinatorially with the Drifter and Fish-hook transcription factors to control midline glial transcription. Postembryonically, *single-minded* is expressed in the brain, including a group of neurons in the central complex that coordinate locomotion. Analysis of adult behavior using a *single-minded* temperature sensitive mutant shows defects in courtship and walking. Mutant flies only walk in circles—they can turn either left or right, but not both. Current work is focused on identifying genes that mediate CNS midline cell fate development, and understanding how Single-minded: Tango interacts with additional regulatory proteins to control their expression.

PAS Proteins. Single-minded, along with Arnt and Period, constitute the founding members of the PAS protein family. PAS proteins are found in all organisms, from bacteria to humans. Prokaryotic and plant PAS proteins are commonly environmental sensors that respond to and mediate the effects of changes in light, oxygen levels, redox, and metabolic state. Most animal PAS proteins belong to the bHLH-PAS class of DNA binding proteins. The Markey Trust has an impressive heritage in bHLH-PAS protein discovery and analysis, having sponsored research in our lab and those of Drs. Tessier-Lavigne, Montell, and Semenza. *Drosophila* and mammalian bHLH-PAS proteins control a variety of biological processes, including toxin metabolism, circadian rhythms, vasculogenesis, tissue-specific development, cell migration, and behavior. Clinically, they are important for understanding tumor growth, sleep disorders, birth defects, and obesity. Our lab has discovered or worked on a number of *Drosophila* bHLH-PAS proteins, including Single-minded, Trachealess (tracheal development), Spineless (appendage formation), Similar (response to hypoxia), Cranky, and Tango (dimerization partner for all of the above). This project has allowed us to generalize about the mechanisms of action of invertebrate and vertebrate developmental bHLH-PAS proteins. Given the fundamental role that bHLH-PAS proteins play in the formation of the nervous system and respiratory system in insects, we have begun to look for similar roles in other species. *Drosophila trachealess* is a master regulator of tracheal transcription and development. We have shown that the crustacean, *Artemia*, has a *trachealess* ortholog that is prominently expressed in the epipodal gills. Although the insect trachea and crustacean gills are divergent morphologically, these results suggest that their formation may be controlled by the same regulatory gene. Furthermore, evolutionary analysis of bHLH-PAS gene expression and function in organisms with distinct mechanisms of CNS and respiratory system development and anatomy may provide important insights into organismal evolution.

STRUCTURAL BASIS OF TRANSCRIPTION

Seth A. Darst, Ph.D.
Laboratories of Molecular Biophysics
The Rockefeller University

Transcription is the major control point of gene expression. RNA in all cells is synthesized by a complex molecular machine, the RNA polymerase (RNAP). In bacteria, RNAP comprises a ~400 kDa core (subunit composition alpha$_2$/beta/beta'/omega), conserved from bacteria to man. Promoter-specific initiation requires additional proteins. In bacteria, a single polypeptide, the sigma factor, binds core RNAP to form holoenzyme.

Our goal is to understand the mechanism of transcription and its regulation. Our approach is to use a combination of structural and biophysical methods spanning resolution ranges (low-resolution: cryo-electron microscopy [EM]; medium: cross-linking analysis and X-ray crystallography; high: X-ray crystallography), complemented by the wealth of functional information already available, to determine the structure/function relationship of RNAP and its complexes with nucleic acids and regulatory factors. Our focus is on the bacterial RNAPs as a model for the cellular RNAPs in general.

Low-resolution EM structures (25-12 Å) of RNAP revealed a molecule shaped like a crab-claw, with a groove or channel for accommodating double-helical DNA.[1,2] In the first step towards high-resolution structural analysis of cellular RNAPs, we determined the 3.3 Å-resolution crystal structure of the 380 kDa core RNAP[3,4] from *T. aquaticus* (*Taq*), providing a basis for further structural and functional studies. For example, the path of the transcript RNA and template DNA through RNAP was tracked using crosslink mapping, resulting in a detailed model of the elongation complex.[5] A co-crystal structure of RNAP with rifampicin revealed the mechanism of inhibition by this important antibiotic.[4] The remarkable conformational flexibility of RNAP was analysed by comparing cryo-EM and X-ray results using newly developed computational tools.[2]

Recent progress is highlighted by crystal structures of the 430 kDa *Taq* holoenzyme (alpha$_2$/beta/beta'/omega/sigma) at 4 Å,[6] and a holoenzyme/promoter DNA complex at 6 Å resolution.[7] These results depended on having high-resolution structures of core RNAP[3,4] and sigma factor domains[8] in-hand. These structures provide fundamental insight into sigma/core RNAP interactions and conformational changes to form holoenzyme, holoenzyme recognition of promoters, and sigma's role in melting the DNA to form the transcription bubble. The structures also provide a basis for models of holoenzyme/promoter complexes along the pathway of open complex formation. The new structural information will guide future investigations at an unprecedented level of detail.

Notes

[1]Darst, S. A.; Kubalek, E. W.; Kornberg, R. D. (1989) *Nature* 340:730-732; Darst, S. A.; Edwards, A. M., Kubalek, E. W.; Kornberg, R. D. (1991) *Cell* 66:121-128; Polyakov, A.; Severinova, E.; Darst, S. A. (1995) *Cell* 83: 365-373.

[2]Darst, S. A.; Opalka, N.; Chacon, P.; Polyakov, A.; Richter, C.; Zhang, G.; Wriggers, W. (2002) *Proc. Natl. Acad. Sci.*, in press.

[3]Zhang, G.; Campbell, E.; Minakhin, L.; Richter, C.; Severinov, K.; Darst, S. A. (1999) *Cell* 98:811-824.

[4]Campbell, E. A.; Korzheva, N.; Mustaev, A.; Murakami, K.; Goldfarb, A.; Darst, S. A. (2000) *Cell* 104:901-912.

[5]Korzheva, N.; Mustaev, A.; Kozlov, M.; Malhotra, A.; Nikiforov, V.; Goldfarb, A.; Darst, S.A. (2000) *Science* 289:619-625.

[6]Murakami, K.; Masuda, S.; Darst, S.A. (2002) submitted.

[7]Murakami, K.; Masuda, S.; Campbell, E.A.; Muzzin, O.; Darst, S. A. (2002) submitted.

[8]Campbell, E. A.; Muzzin, O.; Chlenov, M.; Sun, J. L.; Olson, C. A.; Weinman, O.; Trester-Zedlitz, M. L.; Darst, S. A. (2002) submitted.

HIJACKING THE RIBOSOME: STRUCTURAL BASIS FOR TRANSLATION INITIATION IN HEPATITIS C VIRUS

Jennifer A. Doudna, Ph.D.
Molecular Biophysics and Biochemistry
Howard Hughes Medical Institute
Yale University

Initiation of protein synthesis is a key step in the control of gene expression in eukaryotes. In most cases, recruitment of the 40S ribosomal subunit to a messenger RNA (mRNA) involves recognition of a modified nucleotide cap on the mRNA 5' end by several large translation initiation factors. However, a subset of mRNAs and viral RNAs lack the 5' cap and instead contain a structured RNA element upstream of the coding region called an internal ribosome entry site (IRES) that recruits ribosomes without requiring some or most of the canonical translation initiation factors. In Hepatitis C virus (HCV), the IRES RNA binds directly to the 40S ribosomal subunit and requires just one initiation factor, eIF3, to form a complex primed to initiate translation upon assembly with initiator tRNA and the 60S ribosomal subunit. Images of HCV IRES-40S ribosomal subunit complexes, produced by cryo-electron microscopy in collaboration with J. Frank and C. Spahn, revealed a pronounced IRES-induced conformational change that clamps the 40S subunit on the viral message. This observation together with binding and translation assays suggests that the IRES RNA actively recruits and positions ribosomes during viral infection. Ongoing work focuses on cryo-EM structure determination of the complete HCV IRES preinitiation complex. We have also recently solved a high-resolution crystal structure of the IRES region containing the eIF3 binding site, providing a basis for understanding the role of eIF3 during initiation as well as a target for anti-viral drug design. Ultimately, we hope to elucidate a detailed mechanism for IRES-mediated translation initiation and to use structural data in the design of small molecule inhibitors of the HCV virus.

THE COMPLEX INTERPLAY OF MICROBIAL PATHOGENS WITH EUKARYOTIC CELLS

Joanne Engel, M.D., Ph.D.
Department of Medicine Division of Infectious Disease
University of California, San Francisco

My laboratory is interested in understanding and exploiting the complex interplay of microbial pathogens with eukaryotic cells. One project focuses on how *Pseudomonas aeruginosa* (PA), an important opportunistic pathogen of man, injures epithelial cells. This nosocomial gram negative bacterium is the leading cause of bacteremia and sepsis in patients receiving cytotoxic chemotherapeutic agents, the most common cause of nosocomial pneumonia, a killer of neutropenic and burn patients, the most common cause of corneal ulcers, and a contributing factor to severe pulmonary damage and consequent death in patients afflicted with cystic fibrosis. The virulence potential of PA is exacerbated by the rapid rate at which it develops drug resistance. Indeed, many clinical isolates are insensitive to most or all antibiotics, making the identification of new targets for diagnosis, therapy, and prevention essential for our ability to control this important nosocomial pathogen. Unraveling the complex interactions between PA and its host eukaryotic cells will lead to novel insights into how bacteria attack host cells and outmaneuver the immune system.

A critical determinant of PA infections is the requirement for pre-existing epithelial cell damage. Upon binding, this organism secretes a diverse array of virulence factors that lead to further tissue damage and dissemination. In a novel genetic screen designed to identify new virulence factors required for epithelial cell injury, we demonstrated a key role for the type III secretion system and its secreted effector molecules ExoU and ExoT. In a retrospective clinical study, we have shown that the presence of a functional type III secretion system correlates with outcome in ventilator-associated pneumonia. Such studies suggest that the type III secretion system may be a novel target for intervention in hospitalized patients with PA pneumonia. In addition, we have found that type IV pili are required for type III secretion and for virulence in vitro and in vivo. Using confluent MDCK cells as a model system for an epithelial monolayer, we have shown that the differentiation state of the monolayer affects the ability of PA to damage or enter epithelial cells.

ExoU is a novel cytotoxin that is directly translocated by the type III secretion system from the bacterium to the host cell where it induces necrosis of the host cell. It is required for full virulence in a mouse model of acute pneumonia. In addition to ExoU-mediated necrosis, PA can induce apoptosis in epithelial cells and macrophages. This process requires a functional type III secretion system and appears to work through the Fas pathway. Macrophages isolated from Fas receptor or Fas ligand-defective mice are resistant to PA-induced apoptosis. We are currently carrying out genetic screens to identify the bacterial molecule(s) required for induction of host cell apoptosis.

Using a combination of bacterial genetics and cell biology, we have shown that PA can modulate host cell signaling cascades to regulate its entry into host cells using pathways that are dependent upon the polarization state of the epithelium and that are upregulated in wounded epithelium. In injured or poorly polarized epithelial cells, binding of PA activates Rho GTPase, resulting in bacterial internalization. As epithelial cells regenerate an intact mucosal barrier, they become resistant to PA injury and internalization by downregulation of the entry pathway. These observations begin to explain why PA is such an effective pathogen in the setting of epithelial cell injury.

In addition, this organism can modulate its entry by directly translocating into the host cell cytoplasm the type III secreted effector ExoT, which we have shown to act as a GTPase activating protein towards Rho, Rac, and CDC42. A second domain of ExoT has homology to ADP ribosyl transferases and is required for full activity of ExoT. In addition to its role as an anti-internalization factor, we have shown that ExoT possesses other important physiological activities: it prevents wound healing, disrupts the host actin cytoskeleton, and is required for full virulence in a mouse model of acute pneumonia. Identification of its eukaryotic host cell targets is under way.

Together these studies illustrate the power of combining bacterial genetics with host cell biology. We are currently focusing on understanding (i) the pathways by which ExoT alters the host cell cytoskeleton, (ii) the mechanism of Type III secretion dependent apoptosis, (iii) the role of type IV pili in type III secretion, and (iv) the signal transduction pathways that allow the bacterial pili to respond to environmental signals.

GENETICS OF MALARIAL INFECTION IN MICE

Simon Foote, Ph.D., Vikki Marshall, Rachel Burt, Tracey Baldwin, James Wagglen, and Enmoore Lin
The Walter and Eliza Hall Institute of Medical Research
Melbourne, Australia

There are well-documented associations between host genetics and response to infection in humans. These are most evident in the case of malaria, where many genetic diseases involving the red blood cell are found in geographic coincidence with malarial endemnicity. While association with diseases is relatively straightforward, analysis of other genetic resistance factors which are not so obvious in homozygotes are difficult in human populations. We have elected to use mouse models to study the genetically determined response in mice in an attempt to identify pathways that may be involved in the regulation of the pathophysiological consequence of disease in humans.

We have mapped three loci in murine intercrosses which control various aspects of malarial infection. Two loci, *Char1* and 2 control both outcome to infection and peak parasitaemia levels and *Char3* controls clearance of parasites from the circulation. We have generated congenic mice for each locus and identified minimal congenic intervals still retaining a phenotype distinguishable from the backcross parental line.

A BAC map has been generated for *Cha1*. This covers some 3Mb DNA on murine chromosome 9. Approximately 50 percent of this region has been used to generate BAC congenic animals. One line has a malarial phenotype different from the non-transgenic littermates. This line contains two overlapping BACs which have been sequenced and which contain 11 genes. Efforts to subdivide the region using further BAC transgenesis will be discussed.

MECHANISMS AND GENOMIC CONSEQUENCES OF RETROTRANSPOSON TY1 REPLICATION

Abram Gabriel, M.D.
Department of Molecular Biology and Biochemistry
Rutgers University

My laboratory is interested in two general areas associated with the chromosomal biology of the yeast *Saccharomyces cerevisiae*. The first is the replication fidelity of the endogenous retroelement, Ty1. The genome of *S. cerevisiae* contains ~35 copies of Ty1, which replicates in a manner strikingly similar to vertebrate retroviruses. We observed that Ty1 replication is highly error prone with changes occurring at specific terminal locations. Based on this we developed a model for a novel error generating mechanism, and are now using recombinant Ty1 reverse transcriptase to study the biochemical basis for this phenomenon. Additionally, we have generated active site mutations in the Ty1 RT in the three conserved aspartates. One of these mutants is still capable of efficient polymerization although it is incapable of transposition. Using second site suppressor analysis, in vivo examination of replication intermediates, and biochemical studies of the WT and mutant enzymes, we are examining the basis of RT catalysis, and the functional interactions of different regions of the enzyme.

Our second general area of interest is in the relationship of Ty1 to double-strand break (DSB) repair. We observed that under conditions of a potentially lethal HO endonuclease-induced DSB, chromosomal healing could occur by joining of a portion of Ty1 to the two broken ends. This process involves nonhomologous end joining and is distinct from transposition and homologous recombination with endogenous Ty1 elements. Interestingly, this insertional repair is in competition with other break repair processes such as gene conversion, deletion formation, and rearrangements leading to inversions and translocations. We are studying the genetic determinants of this insertion process. We have also observed that other DNA fragments can insert at DSB sites, particularly mitochondrial DNA fragments. We are investigating the factors that influence the type of insertion event and the ratio of insertions to other repair mechanisms.

GENETIC BASIS OF SUDDEN CARDIAC DEATH AND OTHER CHANNELOPATHIES

Alfred L. George, Jr., M.D.
Division of Genetic Medicine
Vanderbilt University

Ventricular arrhythmias are the single most important cause of sudden cardiac death (SCD) among adults living in industrialized nations. Evidence now exists indicating that genetic factors have a substantial influence in determining population-based risk for SCD and may also account for interindividual variability in susceptibility.

Specific genes underlying various Mendelian disorders associated with inherited arrhythmia susceptibility have been identified. The most well studied familial arrhythmia syndrome is the congenital long QT syndrome (LQTS), an inherited condition of abnormal cardiac excitability characterized by prolongation of the QT interval on surface electrocardiograms of affected individuals. A long QT interval correlates with prolongation of the ventricular action potential owing to delayed myocardial cell repolarization, an arrhythmia-prone cellular substrate. Many LQTS subjects harbor mutations in *SCN5A* encoding the cardiac voltage-dependent sodium channel. Another inherited cardiac arrhythmia, Brugada Syndrome, and certain forms of familial cardiac conduction system disease are also caused by mutations in *SCN5A*. These syndromes join a rapidly growing list of inherited disorders caused by mutations in genes encoding ion channels: the channelopathies.

We have been very successful in characterizing the molecular and biophysical defects caused by mutations in human voltage-gated sodium channels. Our studies utilize recombinant human sodium channels expressed heterologously in cultured cells and interrogated using electrophysiological tools such as the patch-clamp technique. In LQTS, mutations in *SCN5A* result in sodium channels that fail to "close" completely after activating. This functional defect leads to increased sodium influx into myocardial cells, delayed repolarization and increased susceptibility to triggered arrhythmias. By contrast to this "gain-of-function" disturbance in LQTS, sodium channel mutations in Brugada syndrome lead to loss-of-function and electrical imbalances (heterogeneity of repolarization) in the ventricular myocardium that predisposes to arrhythmias. Recently, we have characterized novel *SCN5A* mutations associated with familial cardiac conduction system disease that exhibit a curious combination of gain and loss of function characteristics that account for myocardial conduction slowing. Our studies have helped discern the molecular genotype-phenotype relationships among these three distinct cardiac disorders and have contributed to improved diagnosis and therapy of cardiac arrhythmias.

Our work on the cardiac channelopathies is representative of other investigations into the molecular genetic basis of a variety of other familial disorders affecting muscle contraction (myotonia, periodic paralysis) and associated with epilepsy that have been the focus of my laboratories' research effort.

REGULATION OF MACROPHAGE GENE EXPRESSION BY NUCLEAR HORMONE RECEPTORS

Christopher K. Glass, M.D., Ph.D.
Division of Cellular and Molecular Medicine
University of California, San Diego

My laboratory is interested in how members of the nuclear receptor gene family regulate macrophage development and function. Nuclear receptors are transcription factors that positively or negatively regulate gene expression in response to the binding of small molecular weight ligands. The human genome contains 48 members of this family that include receptors for steroid and thyroid hormones, vitamins, and metabolites of cholesterol and fatty acids. In addition to playing critical roles in the regulation of development and homeostasis, nuclear hormone receptors have been important targets for drug development. Examples include the development of synthetic glucocorticoids for treatment of inflammation and selective estrogen receptor modulators (SERMs) for treatment of breast cancer. Because the transcriptional functions of nuclear receptors can be switched on and off in vitro by addition of small molecules, these proteins have also provided some of the most powerful models for mechanistic studies of transcription. The nuclear receptor field thus spans an extraordinarily broad spectrum of investigation that ranges from basic lines of biochemical, cellular and molecular inquiry to clinical trials of new drugs in major human diseases such as diabetes and atherosclerosis. Owing to the potential medical importance of novel ligands for nuclear hormone receptors, they are the focus of intensive investigation by pharmaceutical companies, biotechnology companies, and academia.

Studies from my laboratory led to the discovery that many members of the nuclear receptor family bind to DNA recognition elements in target genes as heterodimers with retinoid X receptors (RXRs). More recently we have defined coactivators and corepressors that interact with nuclear receptors to mediate their transcriptional effects and have participated in collaborative studies leading to crystal structures of nuclear receptor/ coactivator complexes. Currently, we are focusing on defining the biological roles of the peroxisome proliferator activated receptor γ (PPAR γ) in macrophages. Several lines of evidence indicate that PPAR γ is required for fat cell development and that it regulates glucose homeostasis. PPAR γ has proven to be the molecular target of thiazolidinediones (TZDs), a class of insulin sensitizers that are in clinical use for the treatment of type 2 diabetes mellitus. Approximately three years ago, we reported that high levels of PPAR γ were also expressed in macrophages and that TZDs could inhibit the expression of pro-inflammatory genes. In a follow-up series of studies, we demonstrated that PPAR γ was also highly expressed in macrophage-derived foam cells of human atherosclerotic lesions and that TZDs dramatically reduced the development of atherosclerosis in hypercholesterolemic mice. However, several lines of evidence indicate that despite the net antiatherogenic effect, currently available TZDs also exert pro-atherogenic effects on a subset of macrophage target genes. These findings are of substantial clinical interest, because millions of patients with type 2 diabetes are at markedly increased risk of developing atherosclerosis and its clinical complications. These observations highlight the importance of defining the molecular mechanisms responsible for biological effects of synthetic nuclear receptor ligands and the potential to use this knowledge for the development of selective modulators of nuclear receptor function that are optimized for specific therapeutic outcomes.

SODIUM CHANNELS AND CNS DISEASE

Alan L. Goldin, M.D., Ph.D.
Department of Microbiology and Molecular Genetics
University of California, Irvine

We are studying the effects of mutations in the voltage-gated sodium channel to determine how specific alterations in channel function result in disease in the CNS, using three approaches. In the first part of our studies, we have examined the effects of a missense mutation in the mouse *Scn8a* gene encoding the $Na_v1.6$ sodium channel, which is broadly distributed in brain and spinal cord. The mutation, termed jolting, causes cerebellar ataxia. It results in substitution of threonine for a conserved alanine in the cytoplasmic S4-S5 linker of domain III. Introduction of the mutation into the orthologous rat brain sodium channel shifted the voltage-dependence of activation by 10 mV in the depolarizing direction without any significant changes in the kinetics of either inactivation or recovery from inactivation. The shift in the voltage-dependence of activation observed for the mutant channel would reduce the spontaneous activity of Purkinje cells and lead to a decrease in output from the cerebellum, which is consistent with the phenotype of cerebellar ataxia observed in jolting mice.

In the second part of our studies, we have constructed transgenic mice expressing a mutation of three residues (GAL 879-881 to QQQ) in the cytoplasmic S4-S5 linker of domain II in the rat $Na_v1.2$ sodium channel. This mutation results in slowed inactivation and increased persistent current. The neuron-specific enolase promoter was used to direct *in vivo* expression of the mutant channel in transgenic mice. Three transgenic lines exhibited seizures, and one line was characterized in detail. The seizures in these mice began at two months of age and were accompanied by behavioral arrest and stereotyped repetitive behaviors. Continuous electroencephalogram monitoring detected focal seizure activity in the hippocampus, which in some instances generalized to involve the cortex. Hippocampal CA1 neurons isolated from presymptomatic mice exhibited increased persistent sodium current that may underlie hyperexcitability in the hippocampus. During the progression of the disorder there was extensive cell loss and gliosis within the hippocampus in areas CA1, CA2, CA3 and the hilus. The lifespan of the mice was shortened and only 25 percent survived beyond 6 months of age. Four independent transgenic lines expressing the wild-type sodium channel were examined and did not exhibit any abnormalities. The transgenic mice provide a genetic model that will be useful for testing the effect of pharmacological intervention on progression of seizures caused by sodium channel dysfunction.

In the final aspect of our studies, we have examined the effects of two mutations in the human *SCN1A* gene encoding the alpha subunit of the $Na_v1.1$ sodium channel. These mutations cause generalized epilepsy with febrile seizures plus (GEFS+). Both mutations change conserved residues in putative voltage-sensing S4 segments, T875M in domain II and R1648H in domain IV. Each mutation was cloned into the orthologous rat channel, $rNa_v1.1$, and the properties of the mutant channels were determined in the absence and presence of the beta1 subunit in *Xenopus* oocytes. Neither mutation significantly altered the voltage-dependence of either activation or inactivation in the presence of the beta1 subunit. The most prominent effect of the T875M mutation was to enhance slow inactivation in the presence of beta1, with small effects on the kinetics of recovery from inactivation and use-dependent activity of the channel in both the presence and absence of the beta1 subunit. The most prominent effects of the R1648H mutation were to accelerate recovery from inactivation and decrease the use-dependence of channel activity with and without the beta1 subunit. The DIV mutation would cause a phenotype of sodium channel hyperexcitability while the DII mutation would cause a phenotype of sodium channel hypoexcitability, suggesting that either an increase or decrease in sodium channel activity can result in seizures.

A DECADE-LONG JOURNEY ON THE FRONT LINE OF THE HUMAN GENOME PROJECT

Eric D. Green, M.D., Ph.D.
National Human Genome Research Institute
National Institutes of Health

The Human Genome Project and the fruits of its effort are creating a new era in biomedical research. My laboratory has been firmly planted on the front line of this exciting endeavor for the past decade.

Initially, we focused on the systematic mapping and sequencing of human DNA. As a result of our detailed mapping of chromosome 7, this segment of the human genome was among the first to be sequenced in a large-scale fashion. The resulting mapping and sequencing infrastructure provided a powerful foundation for us to then pursue complementary studies in human genetics, in particular those aiming to identify genes implicated in human disease. Projects within my laboratory led to the identification of the genes responsible for Pendred syndrome (a deafness/goiter disorder), cerebral cavernous malformations (an inherited vascular disease), and an elusive tumor suppressor gene on chromosome 7q31. These studies vividly illustrated how the availability of genome mapping and sequencing data greatly accelerates the process of elucidating the genetic bases of human disease.

Most recently, my laboratory has developed a major program in comparative genomics. As a complement to whole-genome sequencing efforts, we are sequencing the same set of targeted genomic regions in >20 vertebrates. Specifically, large (~250-6,000 kb) chromosomal segments of particular biomedical interest are being isolated in overlapping bacterial artificial chromosome (BAC) clones from multiple species (to date including several non-human primates, ~8 other placental mammals, a marsupial, a monotreme, a bird, and several fish species). The mapped clones are then being sequenced, with the resulting data subjected to rigorous computational analyses. Together, our program is generating >125 Mb of comparative sequence data per year. Importantly, this unique sequence resource is facilitating the development of new computational tools for multi-species sequence comparisons, is revealing the benefits of sequencing species from a range of evolutionary distances, and is serving an important reconnaissance function that should help guide the selection of additional organisms for whole-genome sequencing.

In summary, our decade-long journal along the main trails of the Human Genome Project has allowed us to make important contributions towards the mapping and sequencing of the human genome, towards utilizing the resulting data for studies in human genetics, and, most recently, towards the exploration of myriad genomes in an evolutionarily-deep fashion for the purposes of unraveling the complexities and evolution of the vertebrate genetic blueprint.

NUCLEAR POSITIONING AND CONTROL OF DIVISION AXIS DURING MORPHOGENESIS IN *C. ELEGENS*

Dan Starr, Zhe Chen, and Min Han, Ph.D.
Howard Hughes Medical Institute
University of Colorado

Research in our laboratory aims at understanding the mechanisms of cell differentiation, cell migration, and tissue morphogenesis in *C. elegans*. Two representative projects involving nuclear movement/anchorage and morphogenesis are summarized below.

Nuclear position and migration within a cell are important for cell function in the growth and development of a wide variety of eukaryotes. Our genetic and molecular analyses of the *unc-83*, *unc-84* and *anc-1* genes have revealed protein functions at the nuclear membrane that are involved in nuclear migration and anchorage. UNC-84, a nuclear membrane protein, recruits UNC-83 and ANC-1 protein to the nuclear membrane where they function in nuclear migration and anchorage, respectively. Our results also indicate that ANC-1, a novel and giant coiled-coil protein, may directly mediate nuclear anchorage through a tethering mechanism. UNC-83, expressed at the nuclear envelope of specific cells with migrating nuclei, possibly facilitates migration partly by competing with ANC-1 for UNC-84 binding.

The last round of vulval cell division, particularly the characteristic change of division axis of specific cells is considered an early landmark of vulval morphogenesis. Analysis of *nhr-25* and *lin-40* mutants indicated that they control the asymmetry of vulval cells and proper execution of the division pattern. The *nhr-25* gene encodes a homologue of *Drosophila* Ftz-F1 and mammalian SF-1 NHR proteins. An *nhr-25* mutation that disrupts the DNA-binding activity of the protein specifically blocks the division in cells where the division axes normally change to an orientation perpendicular to that in previous divisions and causes abnormal gene expression in these cells. In addition, the *nhr-25* mutation leads to defects in cell migration and fusion that occur during vulval organogenesis. In contrast, mutations in *lin-40*, which encodes a homolog of MTA, do not block cell division but prevent the change of division axes for the same set of cells. We propose that *lin-40* acts to impose a pause in cell cycle to allow the change of the division axis, while *nhr-25* acts to initiate cell division with a new axis.

A ROLE FOR γδ T CELLS IN TISSUE REPAIR

Wendy L. Havran, Ph. D., Julie Jameson, Stephanie Rieder, and Richard Boismenu
Department of Immunology
The Scripps Research Institute

The focus of my laboratory is to determine the antigen specificity and function of epithelial resident γδ T cells. These cells appear to recognize and respond to self antigens expressed after malignancy, infection or trauma of neighboring epithelial cells. We have demonstrated that after antigen recognition, the epithelial γδ T cells uniquely produce tissue specific cytokines, secrete chemokines and lyse damaged epithelial cells. This data supports a unique role for epithelial γδ T cells in immune surveillance, wound repair, and protection from malignancy.

T cells bearing invariant γδ T cell antigen receptors (TCR) localize to distinct epithelial sites in the adult mouse. The Thy-1⁺ dendritic epidermal T cells (DETC) express a monoclonal Vγ3Vδ1 TCR that is not found elsewhere. We have demonstrated that the DETC recognize and respond to self antigens expressed by neighboring keratinocytes after damage or disease. This antigen recognition is mediated by the DETC γδ TCR. Interestingly, DETC do not express coreceptors CD4 or CD8 and do not express the costimulatory receptor CD28. This may mean that other unidentified molecules play similar roles in DETC activation. Studies in progress are directed towards identification of coreceptors and costimulatory molecules important for DETC function. Recent data from other groups have demonstrated that DETC can specifically kill skin tumor cells through recognition of particular costimulatory molecules. New molecules that are identified may be potential targets for immunotherapy.

Little is known about the specificity and function of T cells that reside in epithelial tissues. Our data supports the idea that these cells recognize a tissue specific self-antigen expressed after epithelial distress. We have demonstrated a new functional role for epithelial-resident γδ T cells in epithelial homeostasis and tissue repair that is distinct from roles played by lymphoid αβ and γδ T cells. We have performed wound healing studies and found defects in keratinocyte proliferation and tissue reepithelialization in the absence of DETC. The mechanism of the DETC effect is through local production of the potent epithelial mitogens KGF-1 and KGF-2. Production of KGFs is a specialized feature of activated epithelial γδ T cells and other T cells do not produce these factors. We also have data in a mouse model of ulcerative colitis demonstrating that intestinal intraepithelial γδ T cells play a role in disease severity and tissue repair that is mediated in part by KGF. Patient studies also suggest a role for resident γδ T cells in epithelial inflammatory disease and malignancy. Identification of molecules involved in DETC activation is an important and necessary step in fully understanding the physiological role played by these cells. The DETC are the prototypic epithelial γδ T cell. As such, information gained in understanding properties of antigen recognition of the DETC may be applicable to other populations of γδ T cells. Costimulatory molecules expressed by αβ T cells have been identified as important targets for immunotherapy, raising the possibility of similar roles for molecules expressed by γδ T cells. Information obtained by these studies may also be useful in design of new treatment strategies for malignancy.

MOUSE MODELS OF X-LINKED DEVELOPMENTAL DISORDERS

Gail E. Herman, M.D., Ph.D.
Division of Molecular and Human Genetics
Children's Research Institute and Department of Pediatrics
The Ohio State University

My laboratory uses genetic approaches to try to understand the basis for selected inherited developmental disorders. Because many of these human disorders are extremely rare and genes on the X chromosome are generally conserved among all mammals, we have focused on X-linked disorders where we study a human disease using a mouse model that often has the same phenotype. Currently, we are studying three groups of disorders in the laboratory, each of which is discussed briefly below.

X-linked dominant male lethal disorders: Recently, my laboratory identified genes responsible for 2 X-linked dominant male lethal disorders in mouse and human. The disorders produce skeletal, skin, and eye abnormalities and involve sequential steps in the cholesterol biosynthetic pathway. Cholesterol levels in affected male mouse embryos at the time of death are normal, suggesting that the pathogenesis of the male lethality must be caused by another mechanism. Placentas from affected male embryos are smaller than those of normal littermates (p < 0.001), and the labyrinthine layer of the placenta appears thinner, disorganized, and has fewer fetal vessels by PECAM staining. There are also statistically significant differences in placental thickness between affected male and affected female placentas. Since most cells in the female rodent placenta undergo preferential inactivation of the paternal X chromosome, we believe that cells derived from allantoic mesoderm that undergo random X-inactivation are responsible for or contribute to the male lethality. We are currently further investigating the pathogenesis of the defects in affected male and female mice using techniques such as in situ hybridization and microarray expression analysis. We are also pursuing analyses of sterol trafficking and regulation in cultured cells derived from affected male embryos.

X-linked myotubular myopathy (MTM1): This is a rare congenital myopathy that presents with hypotonia and respiratory insufficiency. Many affected patients die or are left ventilator dependent and wheel-chair bound for life. The MTM1 gene was isolated in 1996 by our collaborators and appears to be a lipid phosphatase. We have found mutations in the human gene in over 70 affected boys in the United States and have the largest set of clinical data on long-term survivors in the world. As a result of our studies, we now know that a significant number of boys with this disease develop medical complications involving other organ systems. We have employed the yeast two hybrid system to proteins that interact with the MTM protein and are developing a mouse model for the disorder using homologous recombination.

X-linked neural tube defects: Neural tube defects (NTDs) are the second most common human birth defect. The causes for the majority of NTDs are unknown but likely involve both genetic and environmental factors. We have determined that a transcription factor, *Zic3*, is deleted in an X-linked mouse mutant, Bent tail *(Bn)*, that serves as a model for NTDs. In humans, mutations in ZIC3 are associated with laterality (situs) defects and complex congenital heart disease. We and others have identified similar defects in *Bn* mice. Depending on the exact genetic background, we can separate the NTD and situs phenotypes, and we are now mapping these modifiers in a series of genetic crosses. We are also trying to identify upstream regulators and downstream targets of *Zic3* using promoter constructs in tissue culture and *Xenopus* model systems. The genes identified will be candidates for involvement in human NTDs and/or laterality disorders.

SUPPRESSORS OF CYTOKINE SIGNALING

Douglas J. Hilton, Ph.D.
The Walter and Eliza Hall Institute of Medical Research
The Cooperative Research Centre for Cellular Growth Factors
PO Royal Melbourne Hospital

Suppressor of cytokine signaling-1 (SOCS-1) is an important negative regulator of IFNγ signal transduction. While SOCS1 deficient (SOCS1-/-) mice die before weaning of a severe inflammatory disease, mice lacking both SOCS1 and IFNγ survive normally to adulthood, but succumb to a range of diseases in their second year of life. In addition to an SH2 domain, which regulates interaction with tyrosine phosphorylated signaling proteins such as JAKs, SOCS1 contains a 40 amino acid motif, termed a SOCS box. Biochemical studies have demonstrated that the SOCS box interacts with elongin B and C, suggesting that SOCS proteins act as part of a ubiquitin ligase complex and that the termination of signal transduction by SOCS1 may occur in part by targeting signaling proteins for proteasomal degradation. To test this, we have generated mice (SOCS1$^{\Delta/\Delta}$) in which the SOCS-box of SOCS1 has been specifically deleted. SOCS1$^{\Delta/\Delta}$ mice display a phenotype that is intermediate between SOCS1-/- and wild type mice. SOCS1$^{\Delta/\Delta}$ mice survive weaning but succumb to inflammatory disease at 2 to 6 months of age. In vivo and in vitro, cells from these mice respond to IFNγ for longer than cells from wild type mice, but not for as long as cells from SOCS1-/- mice. This suggests that while important, regulation of protein degradation by the SOCS box is not the only mechanism by which SOCS1 attenuates signaling.

IDENTIFICATION AND ANALYSIS OF A SMALL MOLECULE INHIBITOR OF THE BCL-X$_L$ ANTI-APOPTOTIC PROTEINS

David M. Hockenbery, M.D.
Divisions of Human Biology and Clinical Research
Fred Hutchinson Cancer Research Center

The anti-apoptotic Bcl-2 family of proteins confers cellular resistance to a wide range of apoptotic triggers and multi-drug resistance for cancer cells. We developed a cell-based assay to screen for small molecule inhibitors of Bcl-x$_L$, a closely related homolog of Bcl-2 with available NMR and crystallographically-determined solution structures. Cells with over-expressed Bcl-x$_L$ (5-6 fold) were highly resistant to diverse apoptotic stimuli, including the anti-cancer agents doxorubicin and cisplatin, and tumor necrosis factor. Testing of a library of commercially available small molecules identified several compounds with selective toxicity for cells that highly expressed Bcl-x_L compared to control cells. One of these was antimycin A, a known inhibitor of mitochondrial electron transfer complex III. Inhibitors of electron transport at other sites did not exhibit selective killing of Bcl-x_L-expressing cells.

Using molecular docking analysis, antimycin was predicted to bind at a hydrophobic groove on the Bcl-x_L surface. This groove forms an interaction surface for heterodimerization with Bcl-2 family proteins that possess opposite, pro-apoptotic activity. Physical interaction of antimycin and Bcl-x_L was demonstrated by differential fluorescence spectroscopy and isothermal titration calorimetry, with a Kd ~1 mM. Binding was competitive with a hydrophobic groove-binding peptide from the BH3 domain of the pro-apoptotic Bak protein. Antimycin and a pro-apoptotic BH3 domain peptide both selectively triggered loss of mitochondrial DY_m and swelling in Bcl-x_L-expressing mitochondria. Bcl-2 family proteins form membrane pores in synthetic lipid bilayers, first recognized by the structural similarity of Bcl-x_L to the translocation domain of diphtheria toxin. Pore activity of Bcl-x_L, measured by fluorescent dye leakage from synthetic liposomes, was completely inhibited in the presence of antimycin.

These results demonstrated that small non-peptide ligands can directly influence the function of Bcl-2 proteins. Non-peptidyl compounds related to antimycin may be clinically useful to target drug-resistant tumor cells overexpressing Bcl-x_L. However, the inhibitory effect of antimycin on mitochondrial oxidative phosphorylation would preclude further drug development. Chemical modification of antimycin to create the 2-methoxy derivative resulted in loss of respiratory inhibition with the selective toxicity for Bcl-x_L-expressing cells retained. Furthermore, both antimycin and the 2-methoxy derivative inhibit the pore-forming activity and bind Bcl-x_L with similar affinities. Administration of 2-methoxy antimycin A_1 induced regression of human myeloma tumors grown in nod/scid mice without apparent toxicity.

In order to characterize the molecular interaction between antimycin A and Bcl-x_L in more detail, a series of Bcl-x_L proteins with single amino acid substitutions were made to probe the binding pocket surface. We identified mutations that reduce or eliminate sensitivity to antimycin in cell-based assays without compromising the anti-apoptotic functions of Bcl-x_L. Loss of antimycin sensitivity correlates with a reduced ability of antimycin to bind and inhibit pore activity of the recombinant mutant proteins. X-ray crystallographic structures have been obtained for several antimycin-resistant mutants. Of particular interest, the F146W Bcl-x_L

mutant remains antimycin-sensitive, although without detectable anti-apoptotic activity, therefore suggesting that allosteric regulation or additional functions of Bcl-x$_L$ mediate the effects of antimycin. These studies provide detailed structure-activity relationships that can be used for further refinement of Bcl-x$_L$ inhibitors.

CONTROL OF VERTEBRATE MUSCLE CHARACTER

Simon M. Hughes, Ph.D.
MRC Muscle and Cell Motility Unit and Developmental Biology
Research Centre
King's College London

Skeletal muscle contractile properties are controlled by genetic and environmental factors. We are studying muscle development in the early vertebrate embryo using zebrafish as a model system. We have shown that hedgehog signals from the ventral midline are required for correct slow muscle formation. Hedgehogs act, at least in part, through maintaining expression of myogenic transcription factors of the MyoD family. We are investigating the role of other signals and factors in muscle patterning and growth by using the advantages of zebrafish genetics and the optical clarity of the embryo to permit analysis of the behaviour of living cells in response to manipulations. In later life, electrical activity is a major determinant of muscle fibre character. A second line of work examines how electrical activity regulates muscle fibre size and type in mice. We want to understand how electrical signals are integrated over time and turned into a binary decision controlling gene expression on long timescales. We are investigating the role of MyoD family proteins in adult muscle. Ultimately, we aim to unify our embryonic and adult work to understand how muscle character is controlled.

A PROTEOME-WIDE SCREEN FOR PROTEINS REQUIRED FOR CANCER CELL INVASIVENESS BY HIGH-THROUGHPUT CALI

Daniel Jay, Ph.D.
Department of Physiology
Tufts University School of Medicine

A critical aspect of cancer is that cancer cells invade healthy tissue and metastasize to form secondary tumors. Finding proteins required for cancer cell invasiveness would provide new targets for drugs that would impede the spread of cancer and thus improve patient survival. The success of the Human Genome Project and the emergence of proteomics provide biologists with a large number of candidate proteins of potential disease importance. The major bottleneck is in efficient methods to test the functional relevance of these candidates. Previously, our laboratory developed Chromophore-Assisted Laser Inactivation (CALI) to use dye-labeled non-blocking antibodies and laser light to inactivate proteins in situ to validate their roles in cellular processes of clinical importance. We are now applying CALI to test which of the many proteins in the proteome is required for cancer cell invasiveness. We have coupled a multiplex version of CALI to a high-throughput cellular assay for cancer cell invasiveness and are screening antibody libraries directed against a significant fraction of the proteome. Antibodies that affect invasion upon light irradiation are subsequently used to immunoprecipitate the target antigen for identification by mass spectrometry. This screen is akin to mutagenesis but has the advantages of direct protein validation in cells of disease relevance such a human cancer cell lines. We believe that such a reverse proteomic approach is an efficient route to identifying and validating novel protein targets important for cancer cell invasion. Furthermore these studies establish the paradigm that CALI may be used to generate the "knockdown" of protein function to directly validate proteins for a wide array of cellular processes important in disease.

FUNCTIONAL ARCHITECTURE OF THE MAMMALIAN OLFACTORY SYSTEM

Lawrence C. Katz, Ph.D.
Department of Neurobiology
Howard Hughes Medical Institute
Duke University Medical Center

Insights into the functional representations of odors in mammals have been gleaned largely from 2-deoxglucose studies, which greatly limit the range of experiments. To overcome these limitations, we introduced the use of optical imaging of intrinsic signals to rapidly determine the representations of different odorants in the olfactory bulb. In both rats and mice we found that features predicted by molecular studies—bilateral symmetry, stereotypy between animals—had clear correlates in the functional representation of odorants. We uncovered a clear "odortopic" organization in which small changes in molecular structure resulted in spatial shifts in the ensemble of glomeruli representing an odorant. To examine whether the distinctions observed in glomerular activation patterns could allow behavioral discrimination of closely related odorants, we have combined imaging of enantiomers—molecules which differ only in their ability to rotate light—with behavioral testing. Humans can only distinguish certain enantiomers, but rats reliably distinguished all enantiomers tested. The patterns of glomerular activation reflected this ability: some glomeruli were activated in common by both enantiomers, but others were activated exclusively by one or the other, implying the existence of enantiomer-selective odorant receptors.

The olfactory system has an especially intimate connection to the circuitry involved in learning and memory in the mouse brain. We are interested in the cellular and molecular mechanisms by which behaviorally relevant memories are acquired and stored. Using multiphoton imaging in transgenic mice, we've been able to visualize the structural stability of dendrites in the olfactory bulb of adult mice, and to probe whether learning is accompanied by morphological changes. In other experiments, we've employed a miniature, head-mounted microdrive to record from individual olfactory neurons in awake, behaving animals during and after the acquisition of olfactory memories.

METABOLIC "SWITCHES" IN THE DEVELOPING AND DISEASED HEART: FROM INBORN ERRORS TO THE PPAR GENE REGULATORY PATHWAY

Daniel P. Kelly, M.D.
Center for Cardiovascular Research
Departments of Medicine and Molecular Biology and Pharmacology
Washington University School of Medicine

The energy demands of the postnatal mammalian heart are met by high capacity mitochondrial pathways specialized to oxidize fatty acids to produce energy. In the early phases of this project, the identification and molecular genetic characterization of children with inborn errors in mitochondrial fatty acid oxidation (FAO) provided clues that single gene disturbances in cardiac energy metabolism can lead to heart failure and sudden death. Next, we found that the preference of the normal heart for fat versus carbohydrates as substrate for energy production is dynamically regulated during development and in diverse physiologic contexts. Importantly, in certain common acquired forms of heart disease, such as cardiac hypertrophy due to hypertension or coronary artery disease, the capacity of the myocardium to oxidize fats is dramatically reduced, a metabolic phenotype remarkably similar to that of humans with genetic defects in the mitochondrial FAO pathway. Accordingly, we sought to delineate the molecular regulatory events involved in the physiologic control of mitochondrial energy production. We found that tight coordinate control of mitochondrial FAO enzyme gene expression is orchestrated, in part, by a lipid-activated nuclear receptor transcription factor, the peroxisome proliferator-activated receptor α (PPARα). Physiologic studies of genetically engineered "loss-of-function" and "gain-of-function" mice have demonstrated that PPARα maintains lipid and energy homeostasis in the mammalian heart in the context of diverse physiologic conditions, thus serving as a cellular energy metabolic "stress" factor. Mice lacking PPARα die suddenly following a physiologic stress such as fasting or ventricular pressure overload, a phenotype remarkably similar to that of children with genetic defects in the FAO pathway. The activity of PPARα is modulated by its interaction with the inducible transcriptional coactivator PGC-1. PGC-1 expression is induced in the heart following birth and in response to fasting or exercise, conditions known to trigger increased demands for mitochondrial ATP production. Gain-of-function studies in cardiac myocytes in culture and in transgenic mice have shown that PGC-1 not only activates PPARα but also promotes mitochondrial biogenesis through separate transcriptional regulatory pathways. Thus, the PPAR/PGC-1 complex serves as a master regulator of mitochondrial function in the heart. The expression and activity of the PGC-1/PPARα transcriptional regulatory complex is dysregulated in several common cardiovascular disease states. Pathologic cardiac hypertrophy or reduced oxygen availability, such as occurs with myocardial infarction or congenital heart disease, deactivates PPARα/PGC-1 at both transcriptional and post-transcriptional levels in rodents and humans. Conversely, the activity of PGC-1/PPAR, as a ligand-activated transcription factor, shows promise as a target for novel therapeutic strategies aimed at modulating myocardial metabolism in human disease states such as heart failure, diabetes, and myocardial infarction.

THE GENETIC BASIS OF VERTEBRATE EVOLUTION

David Kingsley, Ph.D.
Department of Developmental Biology
Howard Hughes Medical Institute
Stanford University School of Medicine

Despite great interest in the mechanisms that control the origin of new morphological and physiological traits in animals, we still know relatively little about the number of genetic changes required to evolve new traits, the types of genes involved, and whether evolution proceeds primarily by changes in coding or regulatory regions. To address these questions we have initiated a genome-wide linkage analysis of evolutionary change in fish. Three-spine sticklebacks are small teleost fish that have undergone one of the most recent and dramatic evolutionary radiations on earth. Following the widespread melting of glaciers 10,000 years ago, marine sticklebacks colonized thousands of newly created lakes and streams. Many of the freshwater populations subsequently diverged in response to local environmental conditions, generating a large number of isolated populations with dramatic changes in body size, skeletal armor, feeding modifications, and physiological traits at different locations around the world. Although many of these distinct stickleback populations meet a formal species definition, the reproductive barriers between contrasting fish types can be overcome using artificial fertilization in the laboratory, making it possible to carry out a formal genetic analysis of the mechanisms responsible for evolutionary change in vertebrates.

To take advantage of this system we have built the first genome-wide linkage map of three-spine sticklebacks. We have also collected and set up crosses between diverse types of sticklebacks around North America and Northern Europe, generating a large number of progeny segregating a wide range of interesting differences in body armor, feeding structures, anterior posterior patterning, and temperature and salinity preference. Initial mapping results suggest that many of these traits are controlled by a relatively small number of major chromosome regions. We are currently identifying the genes responsible for evolutionary change within these regions, using many of the same forward-genetic and positional cloning methods we have previously used successfully to identify genes responsible for classical morphological traits in mice. These studies should make it possible to determine the number and type of molecular alterations that underlie evolutionary changes in natural populations. In addition, the thousands of independent lakes represent a large number of independent evolutionary experiments. This will make it possible to test evolution proceeds by similar or different mechanisms when similar fish evolve in independent locations around the world.

DID BLOOD VESSELS EVOLVE FROM BLOOD CELLS?

Mark Krasnow, M.D., Ph.D.
Department of Biochemistry
Howard Hughes Medical Institute
Stanford University School of Medicine

My lab is genetically dissecting the developmental programs that control formation of the tracheal (respiratory) system of Drosophila and the mammalian lung. Both of these organs are vast branching networks of epithelial tubes that serve as portals of oxygen entry and transport in the body. One major difference between them is that in Drosophila the tubes extend throughout the body whereas in mammals the tubes end in the lung and oxygen must be transferred to red blood cells and circulate through blood vessels to reach the rest of the body. Drosophila lack blood vessels, but they do have an open circulatory system in which the heart pumps blood through the body cavity and the blood and blood cells percolate around the tissues.

Genetic studies in a number of labs including my own have demonstrated remarkable parallels between Drosophila and mammals in the genetic programs that control development of the respiratory system, heart, and blood cells. The results imply that the Drosophila and mammalian organs are homologous structures, not just functional analogues as was believed for centuries. But Drosophila lack blood vessels, so how did blood vessels arise during evolution? If blood vessels arose late, how did they acquire their intimate relationship with the lung, and how did blood cells end up inside of the vessels? Recently, we discovered that the Vascular Endothelial Growth Factor (VEGF) pathway, a receptor tyrosine kinase signaling pathway that plays a central role in blood vessel development in mammals, controls blood cell development in Drosophila. I will describe how the Drosophila VEGF pathway controls developmental migrations of blood cells, and how these and other recent results point to an intimate evolutionary and developmental association between blood cells and blood vessels. This leads us to speculate that blood vessels arose from blood cells during evolution of the vascular system.

RNA-PROTEIN INTERACTIONS: ROLE IN THE REGULATION OF ONCOGENE EXPRESSION AND NUCLEAR RECEPTOR ACTION IN HORMONE-DEPENDENT CANCER

Peter J. Leedman, Ph.D.
Western Australian Institute for Medical Research
University of Western Australia

The proliferation of breast and prostate cancer cells is dependent upon a variety of growth factor and hormonal signals. Overexpression of members of the type I family of protein tyrosine kinase growth factor receptors (EGF-receptor and *erb*B-2) plays a critical role in the development of breast and prostate cancer. Estrogens and androgens, acting via nuclear hormone receptors (ER and AR, respectively), are also significant contributors to the proliferation of breast and prostate cancer cells. These growth factor receptors and their signaling pathways as well as the coregulators associated with these nuclear receptors are excellent targets for therapeutics. Interactions between RNA and proteins are recognised as making a major contribution to a variety of cellular processes. The field is expanding rapidly, with therapeutic targeting of RNA-protein interactions a growing industry. In the last few years, my laboratory has focused on the elucidation of novel RNA-protein interactions involving specific growth factor receptors, nuclear receptors and coregulators in breast and prostate cancer, with a view to developing specific modulators of tumor cell growth.

Oncogenes and Breast Cancer. Using yeast three hybrid screening we have cloned proteins from a human breast cancer library that target growth factor receptor RNA. One clone encodes a protein that binds growth factor receptor protein (via a SH2 domain) and also growth factor receptor mRNA (via a novel RNA-binding domain). Functional studies provide a role for these novel RNA-protein interactions in regulating receptor expression. Structural studies are in progress to design novel small organic molecule modulators of the interaction for therapeutics.

The Androgen Receptor and Prostate Cancer. AR mRNA is regulated in a cell-specific and divergent manner in prostate and breast cancer cells. We recently identified novel AR mRNA *cis-trans* interactions in these cells, and found that the AR is a target for a complex of RNA-binding proteins. One of these is HuR, a ubiquitously expressed member of the *Elav/Hu* family of RNA-binding proteins involved in the stabilization of several mRNAs. Poly(C) binding proteins, previously implicated in the control of mRNA turnover and translation, also bind AR mRNA and do so simultaneously with HuR. The functional role of these proteins in the regulation of AR expression in cancer cells is currently under investigation.

Novel RNA Coactivator Binding Proteins. The mechanisms underlying ER-mediated transactivation in human breast cancer cells involve a complex set of interactions between the ER and a variety of coregulators. SRA (steroid receptor RNA coactivator), the only described RNA coactivator, plays an important role in this process, and is aberrantly expressed in human breast cancer cells. SRA contains several stable stem-loops suggesting that it is the target for a variety of other coregulators. For example, SHARP is a potent transcriptional repressor that binds to SRA and represses SRA-potentiated ER transactivation. However, the identity and function of additional SRA-binding proteins, as well as the specific target SRA RNA-binding motifs remain to be clearly elucidated. We recently identified a novel family of SRA-binding proteins with a characteristic RNA-binding motif, which modulate SRA-mediated transactivation. Interestingly, these SRA-binding proteins are predominantly nuclear, consistent with their putative role as regulators of transcriptional coactivation. Determining their role in the regulation of estrogen action in breast cancer cells will be of great interest.

HAIRPIN OPENING AND OVERHANG PROCESSING BY AN ARTEMIS/DNA-DEPENDENT PROTEIN KINASE COMPLEX: ROLES IN V(D)J RECOMBINATION AND NONHOMOLOGOUS DNA END JOINING

Yunmei Ma, Ulrich Pannicke, Klaus Schwarz, and Michael R. Lieber, M.D., Ph.D.
Departments of Pathology and Biochemistry and Molecular Biology
University of Southern California School of Medicine

Mutations in the Artemis protein in humans result in hypersensitivity to DNA double-strand break-inducing agents and absence of B and T lymphocytes (radiosensitive severe combined immune deficiency [RS-SCID]). We have now shown that Artemis forms a complex with the 469 kDa DNA-dependent protein kinase (DNA-PKcs) in vitro and in vivo in the absence of DNA. The purified Artemis protein alone possesses single-strand specific 5' to 3' exonuclease activity. Upon complex formation, DNA-PKcs phosphorylates Artemis, and Artemis acquires endonucleolytic activity on single- to double-strand DNA transitions (including 5' and 3' overhangs, as well as hairpins). Finally, the Artemis:DNA-PKcs complex can open hairpins generated by the RAG complex from a 12/23-substrate pair. Thus, DNA-PKcs regulates Artemis by both phosphorylation and complex formation to permit enzymatic activities that are critical for the hairpin opening step of V(D)J recombination and for all of the 5′ and 3′ overhang processing in nonhomologous DNA end joining.

FLUCTUATIONS IN NEUROTRANSMITTER CONCENTRATIONS IN HUMAN BRAIN DIALYSATES DURING SLEEP OR WAKEFULNESS, DURING EPILEPTIC SEIZURES OR FOLLOWING COGNITIVE CHALLENGE

Nigel T. Maidment, Ph.D.,[1] *I. Fried,*[2] *F. Lopez,*[1] *J. M. Zeitzer,*[3] *E. J. Behnke,*[3] *L. C. Ackerson,*[1] *J. Engel, Jr.,*[3] *and C. L. Wilson*[3]
[1]Department of Psychiatry and Biobehavioral Sciences Neuropsychiatric Institute, UCLA School of Medicine
[2]Division of Neurosurgery, UCLA School of Medicine
[3]Department of Neurology, UCLA School of Medicine

We have applied microdialysis to the measurement of extracellular concentrations of monoamine (dopamine, norepinephrine and serotinin) and amino acid (glutamate, aspartate, GABA, taurine) neurotransmitters in several regions of the human brain. Subjects were epilepsy patients who were candidates for neurosurgical resection of tissue encompassing the seizure focus. The data to be presented was collected during one to three weeks following an initial surgical procedure for implantation of deep EEG electrodes in order to determine the location of the seizure focus. Data were collected during quiet wakefulness and during several stages of sleep, during epileptic seizures, and during performance of cognitive tasks.

Materials and Methods. Each implanted assembly consisted of MRI-compatible, flexible, polyurethane probes with seven 1.5-mm-wide platinum contacts with intercontact separation of 1.5-4 mm. These contacts enabled recording of EEG at various sites along the electrode trajectory. Microdialysis probes and platinum/iridium microwires for single unit recording were inserted through the lumen of these probes. The microdialysis membrane (Cuprophan, 200±15-µm diameter, 10 mm length) protruded 10 mm beyond the EEG probe tip. Two fused silica tubes contained within the membrane were used for inflow and outflow of the dialysate. Electrode assemblies were stereotactically placed with MRI and angiographic guidance. Data described were collected in the amygdala, orbital frontal cortex, and anterior hippocampus.

Phosphate-buffered artificial cerebrospinal fluid (aCSF) (NaCl, 125 mM; KCl, 2.5 mM; NaH2PO4, 0.5 mM; Na_2HPO4, 5 mM; $CaCl_2$, 1.2 mM; $MgCl_2$, 1 mM; ascorbic acid, 0.2 mM; pH 7.3 - 7.4) was perfused through the probes at a flow rate of 1.2 µl/min. Sterile, disposable plastic 3-ml syringes were used for a CSF delivery, driven by a pair of CMA-102 minipumps. Flow was established before placement of the microdialysis probes in the brain, and maintained during application of the head dressing, in the recovery room and on the neurosurgery ward, where collection was started on a half-hour basis, using a CMA automated fraction collector. When a seizure occurred, the collection period was immediately reduced to 5 minutes. The "dead space" in the collection tubing allowed for collection of four 5-minute pre-seizure samples. In cases where there were multiple seizures, continuous 5-minute samples were taken. Similarly, the sampling interval was reduced to 5 or 10 minutes during cognitive tasks or sleep studies. Samples were stored at –80°C prior to analysis by HPLC with fluorometric or electrochemical detection.

Results and Discussion. Transient increases in glutamate, aspartate, GABA and taurine were observed in several brain regions sampled during seizure activity, similar to previous reports in the literature. However, this was not a consistent finding. In many cases seizures produced little or no perturbation of extracellular amino acid levels. Dialysate concentrations of dopamine and serotonin in the amygdala varied with state. Dopamine levels were high during waking and low during all stages of sleep but showed no difference between stages of sleep. On the other hand, serotonin was significantly lower during slow wave sleep than during wakefulness, and lower still in REM sleep. Significant increases in dopamine (but not serotonin) were observed in the amygdala during the transition between quiet waking and performance of a simple cognitive task such as reading and during a task requiring working memory. Furthermore, the time-course of the increase in dopamine during an extended learning task correlated with the learning curve during the task.

These data demonstrate that robust and sustained changes in the concentrations of extracellular monoamine neuromodulators occur in the human brain during different behavioral states that are readily measured by microdialysis. The application of recent improvements in the speed and sensitivity of analytical procedures for measurement of these, and other, neuromodulators/neurotransmitters promises to provide further insights into their role in mediating changes in human behavior.

IDENTIFICATION OF NOVEL PROTEIN-PROTEIN INTERACTION DOMAINS INVOLVED IN CELL SIGNALING AND PROTEIN TARGETING

Benjamin L. Margolis, M.D.
Department of Internal Medicine and Biological Chemistry
Howard Hughes Medical Institute
University of Michigan Medical School

With the sequencing of the human genome complete it becomes increasingly important to understand the role of newly identified but uncharacterized proteins. One mechanism to understand the biological role of proteins is to identify functional domains within the sequence of the proteins. One type of motif found in many proteins is the protein-protein interaction domain. Our laboratory works at defining these domains and trying to understand their biological function in mammalian cells. Presently we are focused on understanding the role of protein-protein interaction domains in signal transduction and protein targeting. Our group identified and has extensively studied a protein-protein interaction domain called the Phosphotyrosine Binding (PTB) domain.

Our initial work showed that proteins such as Shc contain a PTB domain and play an important role in signaling by growth factor receptors. The PTB domain in Shc allows it to bind to tyrosine phoshorylated growth factor receptors and connect certain growth factor receptors to the Ras signaling pathway. More recent work has shown that the PTB domains do not always bind to tyrosine phosphorylated proteins and can interact with proteins in a nonphosphotyrosine dependent fashion. This has led to discoveries by our group and others into the important role of PTB domains in cell signaling, neurological development, and cholesterol homeostasis.

Our most recent work has focused on the PTB domain protein, X11. This protein is the mammalian homologue of the *C. elegans* Lin-10 protein. Work of another Markey Scholar, Stuart Kim, has demonstrated that Lin-10 is complexed with two other proteins Lin-2 and Lin-7 and these proteins are crucial for the targeting of the worm EGF-Receptor to the basolateral surface. Our work has demonstrated a similar complex in mammalian brain and a complex of mLin-2 and mLin-7 in mammalian epithelia. In mammalian epithelia we have found that mLin-2 is not the only partner of mLin-7 but that at least five different proteins can bind mLin-7. Two new proteins we identified that associate with mLin-7 are called Pals for Proteins Associated with Lin-7. By identifying these additional mLin-7 binding partners we have been able to define a new domain in the Pals and mLin-2 proteins that allow them to interact with mLin-7.

We have also demonstrated that this domain is present in the amino-terminus of Lin-7 itself. We call this new domain the L27 domain because we first identified it in Lin-7 and Lin-2 proteins. Proteins like Lin-2 and Pals1 contain two L27 domains, the carboxy-terminal L27 (L27C) domain binds to the L27 domain of mLin-7 whereas the partners of the amino terminal L27 (L27N) domain were unknown. We have been examining the role of the L27N domains in the targeting of the Pals1 protein. We have found that Pals1 is targeted to the tight junction of epithelia cells by the L27N domain and that this domain binds a novel PDZ domain protein called Pals1 Associated Tight Junction Protein (PATJ). Our data finds that Pals1 and PATJ form a tight junction complex in mammalian epithelia that is conserved in Drosophila proteins known to be crucial for epithelial polarity.

GLOBAL GENE EXPRESSION IN SALMONELLA TYPHIMURIUM, AND GENE CONTENT SHARED WITH OTHER SALMONELLA, DETERMINED BY MICROARRAYS

Michael McClelland, Ph.D.,[1] Jonathan Frye,[1] Rick Wilson,[2] Sandy Clifton,[2] John Spieth,[2] Ken Sanderson,[3] Steffen Porwollik[1]
[1]Sidney Kimmel Cancer Center
[2]Genome Sequencing Center, Washington University
School of Medicine
[3]University of Calgary

Following our sequencing of the Typhimurium genome we have arrayed the complete open reading frame set by spotting PCR amplified ORFs on glass slides. We have begun a survey of expression changes in Typhimurium in response to stresses that simulate aspects of the host response to infection, and expression changes induced by mutations of the major known regulators of pathogenesis. In addition, genomes from other Salmonella were hybridized to the array. Despite being closely related, the Salomonella differ widely in host range and pathogenic routes. We present data on the presence and absence of homologues of *S. typhimurium* LT2 genes obtained from members of all seven Salmonella subspecies, and from *Salmonella bongori*. Genes that were acquired during key stages of Salmonella evolution were determined including those gained at the branching point of subspecies I, which contains all the major Salmonella pathogens of warm-blooded animals.

THE MAP OF CHEMICAL SPACE ON THE OLFACTORY BULB

Markus Meister, Ph.D.
Molecular and Cellular Biology
Harvard University

Our nose senses odors using several hundred types of olfactory neu-rons. Each type expresses a distinct receptor protein to bind ligands in the air stream. Neurons of the same type project their axons to the same location in the olfactory bulb, a small ball of fibers ~100 µm across, called a glomerulus. It is now possible to monitor the neural activity in ~200 of these glomeruli simultaneously, through methods of optical recording from the brain surface of anesthetized animals. We have combined this recording method with a stimulating machine that can rapidly deliver ~1000 odors to the animal. In this way, one can measure the sensitivity of 200 olfactory receptor proteins to hundreds of different ligands. This is providing new insight into the affinity spectra of these receptors, the nature of the neural code for smells, and the structure and development of the olfactory bulb.

PROTEOME STARGAZING

Jonathan Minden, Ph.D.
Department of Biological Sciences
Carnegie Mellon University

Proteomics is a new and burgeoning field that has emerged as a major focus since the sequencing of the human genome and the genomes of many other model organisms. The proteome is defined as the collection of proteins found in cells, tissues, and organisms. Individual cells may ex-press 5,000-10,000 different proteins, while a whole organism can express >1,000,000 protein isoforms. One of the main goals of proteomics is to identify protein changes that occur normally during development and tissue differentiation and as a result of disease, drug treatment, and envi-ronmental change. There are two main components to proteomics: sepa-ration of cellular proteins into individual components and identification of the genes that encode individual proteins. Protein separation is usually conducted by two-dimensional gel electrophoresis, which separates pro-teins based on size and charge. Identification of the gene encoding iso-lated proteins is done by mass spectrometry where one compares the mass of specifically-generated protein fragments to a database of predicted protein fragments.

The scale of the genome sequencing projects pales in comparison to the goal of proteome projects. There are plans to search for protein changes in dozens of different tissues at dozens of different stages of development and dozens of different diseases from hundreds of samples and in the presence of thousands of different drugs and conditions. The number of possible experiments is truly staggering. There is great need to increase the rate of proteome analysis 10-100 fold, or more. We have developed a method, called difference gel electrophoresis (DIGE), to rapidly identify protein changes between two or three samples on the same two-dimensional electrophoresis gel. This method relies on fluorescently tagging all proteins in each sample with one of a set of matched fluorescent dyes that do not affect the relative mobility of proteins during electrophoresis. This method greatly reduces the complexity of the search for protein differences from several thousand proteins observed in the protein extract to several dozen candidate proteins that are significantly different between the samples. DIGE is more sensitive than silver staining and can detect changes as little as 0.01 percent of total protein. The imaging system can detect a 10,000-fold range of protein concentrations; silver staining can only detect a 30-fold concentration range. This level of sensitivity and discrimination challenges the performance of mass spectrometers to identify the genes that encode the proteins difference that we can detect using DIGE. This presentation will describe the uses of DIGE and future challenges for proteome analysis.

FUNCTIONAL GENOMIC ANALYSES OF CELLULAR MORPHOLOGY USING HIGH-THROUGHPUT RNAI SCREENS

A. Kiger, [* 1] *B. Baum,* [* 1,4] *S. Armknecht,* [1] *M. Chang,* [1] *S. Jones,* [2]
B. Sönnichsen, [2] *C. Echeverri,* [2] *M. Jones,* [3] *A. Coulson,* [3]
Norbert Perrimon, Ph.D. [1]
[1]Department of Genetics, HHMI/Harvard Medical School
[2]Cenix BioScience GmbH, Dresden
[3]Sanger Centre, Cambridge
[4]Ludwig Institute, University College of London
* These authors contributed equally.

The vast potential of the genome sequence relies on new technologies capable of functional and systematic analyses of the ~14,000 predicted *Drosophila* genes. The use of RNA-interference (RNAi) in *Drosophila* cell cultures by the simple addition of dsRNA to the culture medium provides an effcient method to reduce or eliminate the expression of specific genes, yielding phenocopies of loss-of-function mutations. The availability of predicted gene-specific sequences in combination with RNAi application in cell cultures enables the design of a large-scale approach to study of cell-biological functions. I will describe our efforts at developing high-throughput screens based on RNAi methodology using *Drosophila* cell cultures in 384-well plates and automated microscopic imaging.

In a pilot screen, we assembled a set of 1000 dsRNAs representing genes predicted to encode for regulators central to many fundamental cellular processes, including all the small GTPases and GTPase regulators, kinases, and phosphatases. We screened this collection for genes that alter cell morphology and cytoskeletal organization in different *Drosophila* cell lines. With analysis of actin filaments, microtubules, and DNA, we were able to visibly distinguish phenotypic classes that revealed specific functions associated with specifc members within each gene family. The identification of all the dsRNAs that shared similar phenotypes revealed genes that delineate specific pathways that affect cell form and function. To identify additional components in the pathway, we carried-out RNAi modifier screens. By using RNAi as a screening tool we have been able to identify functions for specific GTPases and associated pathways.

CATHEPSIN B: A NOVEL DRUG TARGET FOR TOXOPLASMOSIS

Sharon Reed, M.D.
Department of Pathology and Medicine
University of California, San Diego

Toxoplasmosis is one of the most common parasitic infections of man, with infection rates approaching 90 percent in some countries. Although the majority of patients have asymptomatic, dormant infection for life, serious complications result from congenital infection or reactivation disease in immunocompromised patients, particularly with AIDS. *Toxoplasma gondii* encephalitis is the most common cause of central nervous system infection in patients with AIDS and is uniformly fatal unless diagnosed and treated early. Current treatment regimens are often limited by toxic side effects of the drugs. Thus, further understanding of the pathogenesis of infection by *T. gondii* and the identification of potential drug targets is critical.

Cysteine proteinases play a key role in a number of host-parasite interactions and can be targeted by specific inhibitors. We have cloned a cathepsin B gene, TgCP1, from *T. gondii.* The enzyme contains a classic pre-pro sequence, an active site triad, and dipeptidyl carboxypeptidase activity characteristic of cathepsin B's of higher eukaryotes. When models of the *T. gondii* enzyme were compared to human and rat cathepsin B, a high degree of similarity between the active site regions was found. The structure of the enzyme predicts substrate specificity for positively charged amino acids, which was confirmed with both purified native and active recombinant enzyme.

Cathepsins in higher eukaryotes are located in acidic lysosomes, where they play an important role in protein processing and breakdown. Classic lysosomes are not detected in toxoplasma. Instead, TgCP1 localizes to the rhoptry, a unique club-shaped organelle at the apical end of the parasite. Rhoptries are critical for host cell invasion and are packaged with specialized hydrolases, cholesterol, and membranes for secretion, characteristic of lysosomal-like organelles. All rhoptry proteins are synthesized as prepro-proteins, which must be processed to their active form. We found that specific cathepsin B inhibitors blocked the processing of ROP2, suggesting that it was involved in rhoptry protein processing. When specific inhibitors were added to infecting parasites, invasion of host cells was blocked. If cell-permeable inhibitors were added after infection was initiated, significantly fewer host cells were infected. These findings suggest that specific inhibitors may block both invasion and intracellular survival of the parasite.

In future studies, we plan to evaluate the role of TgCP1 in parasite survival using specific inhibitors and anti-sense RNA, crystallize the enzyme for drug modeling to identify novel new drugs, and test these compounds in animal models of infection. These studies should not only provide important information about the pathogenesis of one of the most serious opportunistic infections of AIDS patients, but could also establish a role for cysteine proteinase inhibitors as novel new therapeutic agents for toxoplasmosis.

DEFINING THE FUNCTIONS OF HNRNP PROTEINS USING GENOMICS AND DROSOPHILA GENETICS

Marco Blanchette, Emmanuel Labourier, and Donald Rio, Ph.D.
Department of Molecular and Cell Biology
University of California, Berkeley

Alternative splicing is a strategy that eukaryotic cells have evolved to generate multiple protein isoforms from a single gene. Computer analysis of the human genome predicts that 40 to 60 percent of all genes undergo alternative splicing. Despite the fact that the biochemistry of the spliceosome is well understood, little is known about the mechanism governing alternative splice site selection. The *Drosophila* hrp48 and PSI genes encode RNA binding proteins structurally related to the mammalian hnRNP (heterogeneous nuclear ribonucleoprotein) A/B and hnRNP K proteins, respectively. HnRNP proteins are a large family of nucleic acid binding proteins involved in many essential cellular processes, such as alternative pre-mRNA splicing regulation, RNA stability, RNA transport, translational regulation, as well as telomere maintenance and transcriptional regulation. Previous studies have shown that hrp48 and PSI are involved in the soma-specific inhibition of the P-element transposase third intron pre-mRNA splicing. In addition to their roles in the regulation of P-element transposase expression, both hrp48 and PSI play other essential functions in *Drosophila* since mutant hrp48 and PSI strains exhibit larval lethality. Identification of cellular RNAs bound by both proteins will help to clarify their cellular functions. Using high density cDNA microarrays, a genome-wide search for PSI and hrp48 RNA target has been performed. Briefly, hrp48- or PSI-containing ribonucleoprotein particles were purified from embryonic nuclear extracts using gradient sedimentation and immunoaffinity chromatography. The protein-associated RNAs were then extracted, reverse-transcribed, labeled and hybridized to *Drosophila* cDNA microarrays representing more than 5000 different genes. Using this approach, several putative targets have been identified for both hrp48 and PSI. Using Drosophila strains expressing a mutant form of the PSI protein, we have found that alternative splicing of one such target, the sqd/hrp40 gene was affected in the PSI mutant. We are currently in the process of developing in vitro assays to address how PSI controls alternative splicing of the sqd pre-mRNA. We are also investigating if expression or processing of some of the hrp48 target RNAs are affected in an hrp48 mutant genetic background. The splicing pattern of intron-containing targets will be assayed by RT-PCR experiments while the level of mRNA expression is being tested using cDNA microarrays. Finally, we will look at the cellular localization of the putative hrp48-regulated target RNAs in the RNA interference hrp48-disrupted cells using whole mount embryo in situ hybridization. Together, these molecular genetic analyses and the identification of putative hrp48- and PSI-regulated cellular target RNAs will help to understand the roles these RNA binding protein in play for *Drosophila* mRNAs. More generally, these studies will give us tools to explore how these classes of hnRNP proteins function in RNA processing, transport and/or stability.

HYPOXIA-INDUCIBLE FACTOR 1: MASTER REGULATOR OF OXYGEN HOMEOSTASIS IN HEALTH AND DISEASE

Gregg L. Semenza, M.D., Ph.D.
McKusick-Nathans Institute of Genetic Medicine
The Johns Hopkins University School of Medicine

Hypoxia-inducible factor 1 (HIF-1) is a global regulator of O_2 homeostasis that activates the transcription of >50 known target genes encoding proteins which mediate cellular adaptation to O_2 deprivation (via induction of glycolytic metabolism and growth factor signaling pathways) or increased O_2 delivery (via regulation of the erythroid, cardiac, vascular, and respiratory systems). Progress in elucidating the mechanisms and consequences of HIF-1 activity since our isolation of the factor in 1995 is summarized below.

Mechanism of O_2-regulated HIF-1α activity. HIF-1α is a heterodimer consisting of a constitutively-expressed HIF-1β subunit and a HIF-1α subunit, the expression of which is determined by the cellular O_2 concentration. HIF-1α is modified by prolyl hydroxylases (PHs) which require O_2 at concentrations that are rate-limiting under physiologic conditions. The von Hippel-Lindau tumor suppressor protein (VHL) binds to HIF-1α only when the protein has been prolyl-hydroxylated and targets it for ubiquitination and proteasomal degradation. In addition to the regulation of HIF-1α protein expression, the transcriptional activity of HIF-1α is also negatively regulated under normoxic conditions by interactions with VHL and the corepressor FIH-1α, which both recruit histone deacetylases to HIF-1, thus providing a molecular basis for the regulation of gene expression by HIF-1 in response to changes in cellular oxygenation.

Consequences of HIF-1 deficiency in knockout mice. Analysis of knockout mice has revealed that HIF-1α expression is required for embryogenesis. HIF-1α–null mice die at midgestation with neural tube defects, cardiac and vascular defects, and massive mesenchymal cell death. Mice that are heterozygous for the null allele develop normally and are indistinguishable from their wild-type littermates under normoxic conditions. When wild-type mice are subjected to chronic hypoxia, they develop pulmonary vascular remodeling and right ventricular hypertrophy. These responses are markedly impaired in the heterozygotes, implicating HIF-1α in the pathogenesis of pulmonary hypertension, a lethal complication of chronic lung disease. The heterozygous mice also have ventilatory abnormalities due to a failure of the carotid body chemoreceptors to sense and/or respond to hypoxia.

Role of HIF-1 in angiogenesis. Among the targets regulated by HIF-1 is the gene encoding vascular endothelial growth factor (VEGF) which plays a critical role in angiogenesis. Pre-clinical trials of therapeutic angiogenesis utilizing VEGF gene therapy for ischemic disorders indicate that VEGF stimulates neovascularization but that the resulting vessels have excessive permeability. In contrast, increased HIF-1α expression results in increased vessels with normal permeability. These results suggest that HIF-1α controls the expression of angiogenic factors in addition to VEGF, resulting in a more physiologic outcome. Clinical trials of HIF-1 gene therapy in patients with limb or myocardial ischemia are currently in progress.

Role in HIF-1α in protecting ischemic cells from infarction. In models of myocardial and cerebral ischemia, subjecting animals to brief episodes of ischemia protects against prolonged ischemia 24 hours later that would otherwise result in infarction (delayed preconditioning). Recent studies indicate that HIF-1α activity is required for delayed preconditioning in the heart.

Involvement of HIF-1α in tumor progression. In animal models, genetic manipulations that increase or decrease HIF-1 expression are associated with increased or decreased tumor growth and angiogenesis, respectively. Immunohistochemical analysis of human tumor biopsies has revealed that HIF-1α is overexpressed in common human cancers and their metastases. In brain and breast tumors, HIF-1 expression is correlated with tumor grade and angiogenesis. Studies of oropharyngeal squamous cell cancers, early-stage breast and cervical cancer, and ovarian cancer have demonstrated that increased HIF-1α expression predicts radiation resistance and patient mortality. These studies indicate, first, that the determination of HIF-1α levels at the time of diagnosis may identify patients who require more aggressive therapy in order to survive their disease and, second, that pharmacologic inhibition of HIF-1α activity may be of therapeutic utility. The Developmental Therapeutics Program at the NCI is presently screening for small molecule inhibitors of HIF-1α that can be utilized for proof-of-principle experiments in animal models and as lead compounds for the development of novel chemotherapeutic agents.

Conclusion. Heart disease, cancer, stroke, and chronic lung disease account for two thirds of all deaths in the U.S. Alterations in O_2 homeostasis and HIF-1α expression play major roles in the pathophysiology of these disorders. Genetic or pharmacologic manipulation of HIF-1α activity represents a novel therapeutic approach to these common causes of mortality.

IN VIVO ANALYSES OF T CELL COSTIMULATORY PATHWAYS

Arlene H. Sharpe, M.D., Ph.D.
Department of Pathology and Brigham and Women's Hospital
Harvard Medical School

My research focuses on the in vivo biology of costimulation and its rolein regulating immune responses. Costimulation appears pivotal in determining whether T cell antigen recognition leads to T cell activation or anergy. For antigen-specific T cell activation to occur, two signals are needed. The interaction between the T cell receptor (TCR) complex and antigen-MHC is necessary, but not sufficient for T cell activation. Costimulatory signals, provided cell surface molecules are expressed on antigen-presenting cells, determine the outcome of TCR engagement, since they augment T cell proliferation and effector functions, such as lymphokine production. The interaction between CD3/TCR and antigen-MHC in the absence of costimulation not only results in a failure to induce an immune response, but often also results in functional inactivation of mature T cells, leading to a state of T cell unresponsiveness or death. Thus, T cell costimulatory signals play a critical role in determining the fate of a T cell. Several receptor-ligand pairs, which are primarily either members of the immunoglobulin supergene family or tumor necrosis factor receptor family, have costimulatory function because they induce activated T cells to proliferate after TCR signaling. The B7-CD28/CTLA4 costimulatory pathway appears to be particularly important, because of its unique capacity to prevent the induction of anergy.

The main approach that my laboratory has been taking to analyze the in vivo function of costimulatory pathways is to generate and analyze the immune capabilities of mice lacking costimulatory ligands and receptors using gene targeting approaches. We have focused primarily upon the B7:CD28 superfamily. Our mouse strains have provided a genetic means for dissecting the hierarchy of costimulatory pathways in the development of an immune response. Our studies have revealed striking and unexpected functions of costimulatory pathways. Our studies of B7-1 deficient mice provided the first evidence for the existence of additional functional CD28/CTLA-4 counter-receptors in vivo. As a result of these findings, a second CD28/CTLA-4 counter-receptor, B7-2, was cloned. Our studies revealed that B7-2 is the major early activating costimulator in this pathway. Mice lacking both B7-1 and B7-2 exhibit profound immunologic deficits and have demonstrated a critical role for this pathway in IgG class switching and germinal center formation. Our CTLA-4 deficient mouse revealed a critical role for CTLA-4 in turning off activated T cells and a previously unsuspected means by which costimulation can regulate responses to self antigens and potentially offers new approaches for regulating Tcell activation and tolerance.

There is currently great interest in manipulating costimulatory signals for therapeutic purposes. Specifically, learning how to inhibit costimulatory pathways may enable new methods for achieving tolerance for tissue transplantation and for controlling autoimmune diseases and allergies, whereas learning how to use costimulatory pathways to augment immune responses may lead to new immunization strategies for infectious agents and tumor immunity. Clinical trials using costimulatory blockade to block transplant rejection and ameliorate autoimmune diseases are in progress.

LESSONS FROM ABL: IMPLICATIONS FOR THE FUTURE OF TARGETED CANCER THERAPEUTICS

Richard A. Van Etten, M.D., Ph.D.
Center for Blood Research and Department of Genetics
Harvard Medical School

A new era of targeted cancer therapy was inaugurated in May 2001 with the FDA approval of STI-571 (Gleevec®/imatinib mesylate) for the treatment of chronic myeloid leukemia (CML). STI-571 is a phenylaminopyrimidine compound that is a potent and selective inhibitor of the Abl, PDGFbR, and Kit tyrosine kinases. An ATP mimetic, STI-571 binds to the ATP-binding site of the Abl catalytic domain and effectively inhibits Abl kinase activity in vitro and in vivo at concentrations of 0.1-1.0 mM. In phase I trials, STI-571 was remarkably effective as a single agent in interferon-resistant CML chronic phase patients, inducing durable hematologic remissions in 90 percent and major cytogenetic responses in 55 percent of patients. This agent has already radically altered the way patients with CML are managed, and is being heralded as the paradigm for the development of anti-cancer drugs in the future. From my perspective as a hematologist studying the molecular pathophysiology of leukemia, the STI-571 story raises several important issues: (1) The importance of precise knowledge of molecular drug targets in cancer. Work from our laboratory and many others over the previous decade demonstrated that the Bcr/Abl fusion tyrosine kinase, the product of the Philadelphia chromosome, is the direct cause of CML. Definition of the fundamental genetic abnormalities in cancer cells is a prerequisite to developing targeted therapies. Our work strongly argues that accurate animal models of human cancer are critical to this effort, as results obtained in cultured cells have often been misleading. (2) The remarkable activity of STI-571 in CML as a single agent, and whether this can be generalized to other cancers. Our work suggests that solitary expression of Bcr/Abl in a hematopoietic stem cell is sufficient for induction of CML, and this may account for the extreme sensitivity of this leukemia to STI-571. However, solid tumors may have additional abnormalities in addition to activated tyrosine kinases that contribute to the oncogenic phenotype. Thus, while a subset of gastrointestinal stromal cell tumors that express activated c-Kit tyrosine kinase receptors also respond to STI-571, no complete remissions are observed. Trials of EGFR inhibitors in head and neck and glial tumors are just beginning. (3) Acquired drug resistance is a central problem in cancer therapy, and targeted therapeutics will be no different. Although STI-571 is effective in CML chronic phase, in patients with advanced disease, including accelerated phase, myeloid and B-lymphoid blast crisis, and those with de novo Ph-positive B-lymphoblastic leukemia, STI-571 is less effective. Although 50-70 percent of such patients initially respond to the drug, 60 percent of myeloid blast crisis patients and all B-lymphoid leukemia patients relapse within 3 to 6 months of starting therapy. Our laboratory and others have shown that a major mechanism of resistance is point mutations in the Abl catalytic domain that directly confer drug resistance. (4) Combinations of targeted therapies may be a strategy for improving responses to STI-571 and preventing the development of resistance. By analogy to HIV infection (like CML, another acquired dominant genetic disease of the blood) where treatment targeting both viral reverse transcriptase and protease is more efficacious than monotherapy, it is plausible that targeting critical signaling pathways downstream of Bcr/Abl will synergize with kinase inhibitor therapy. Again, animal models are the best way to validate such pathways. (5) Can the success with STI-571 be repeated? This is a complex question with both scientific and economic/social aspects. The development of STI-571 is often cited as a successful example of high-throughput drug screening and/or rational drug design. Both are incorrect, as the screen that identified the basic pharmacophore of STI-571 used protein kinase C, and the structural basis for the selectivity of action of the compound against Abl is still not understood. In addition, economic forces will play a major role in dictating which drugs will be developed for which diseases. The STI-571 program was nearly cancelled by Novartis less than 18 months before FDA approval due to the small perceived market opportunity, and resurrected only after direct pressure from leukemia patients. There are other leukemias with excellent tyrosine kinase targets for which drug development may never proceed due to the comparatively small number of patients with the disease.

TWO FAMILIES OF BIR-CONTAINING PROTEINS: INHIBITORS OF APOPTOSIS OR REQUIRED FOR MITOSIS

David L. Vaux, Ph.D.
The Walter and Eliza Hall Institute of Medical Research
Melbourne, Australia

Inhibitor of apoptosis (IAP) proteins all bear one or more copies of a motif termed a baculoviral IAP repeat (BIR), a novel zinc finger fold. Certain BIR bearing proteins from baculoviruses, Drosophila and mammals inhibit cell death by binding to processed caspases. The Drosophila IAPs are antagonized by small pro-apoptotic molecules Grim, HID and Reaper. Mammalian IAPs are antagonized by mitochondrial proteins Diablo/Smac and Htra2, which interact via their processed amino-termini. Survivin is a protein that bears a single, structurally distinct BIR, and is expressed in all cancer cells, but is usually undetectable in cells from normal adult tissues. We have identified and deleted surviving homologues in the yeasts *S. pombe* and *S. cerevisiae*, in *C. elegans* and in the mouse. The phenotypes of these mutant organisms, and the pattern of Survivin expression revealed by antibodies, indicates that Survivin, inner centromere protein (INCENP) and aurora kinase 1 and their respective homologues function in concert to coordinate chromosome segregation and cytokinesis. The requirement for Survivin for cell division explains why it is expressed in cancer cells, which are dividing, but not in most normal adult cells, which are not.

A COMMON THEME IN THE PATHOGENESIS OF BACTERIAL INFECTION OF THE HUMAN RESPIRATORY TRACT

Jeffrey N. Weiser, M.D.
Departments of Microbiology and Pediatrics
University of Pennsylvania

Choline, a major component of eukaryotic membrane lipids, has been considered to be a highly unusual feature in prokaryotes. This laboratory has recently shown that choline in the form of phosphorylcholine (ChoP) decorates the oligosaccharide portion of the LPS of *Haemophilus influenzae*. Choline is obtained directly from the airway surface fluid or stripped off of host membrane lipids by a cell-surface glycerophosphodiesterase causing a cytotoxic effect on the ciliated epithelium. A MAb that recognizes ChoP shows that the ChoP epitope is a common feature of other major pathogens that reside primarily on the mucosal surface of the human respiratory tract. In addition to *Streptococcus pneumoniae*, where ChoP has long been recognized as a constituent of its teichoic acids, the ChoP epitope is found on pili of *Neisseria meningitidis* and *gonorrheae*, a temperature regulated cell-envelope protein in *Pseudomonas aeruginosa*, the LPS of commensal Neisseria species and *Actinobacillus actinomycetemcomitans*, and a polar membrane lipid in various mycoplasma species.

The cell-surface expression of ChoP is subject to phase variation at a frequency of 10^{-3}/generation due to slip-stranded mispairing of multiple tandem 5'-CAAT-3' repeats within the open reading frame of the gene expressing choline kinase, *licA*. This suggests that it is not always advantageous for the organism to express ChoP. Our ability to define the genetic basis of choline incorporation in *H. influenzae* has allowed us to compare constitutive ChoP+ and ChoP- phenotypes to demonstrate that on the mucosal surface in both animal models and in human carriage there is strong selective pressure for bacteria expressing ChoP(ChoP+). In contrast, during invasive disease there is a selection for bacteria with an out-of-frame number of 5'-CAAT-3' repeats in *licA*(ChoP- phenotype).

ChoP appears to have multiple effects on the ability of respiratory tract pathogens to interact with their host. ChoP may function in binding and invasion of host cells through mimicry of the natural ligand for the receptor for platelet activating factor (rPAF) expressed on the apical surface of the respiratory epithelium. In addition, ChoP renders the organism more resistant to the bactericidal effects of the antimicrobial peptide LL-37, which is present in airway surface fluid and targets structural differences between host and microbial membranes. In contrast, for some strains ChoP confers sensitivity to killing mediated by the binding of the serum acute phase reactant, C-reactive protein (CRP). Binding of CRP to ChoP causes the activation of the classical pathway of complement by ligation of C1q. In this regard, CRP seems to be a component of innate host defense that specifically targets microbes bearing cell-surface ChoP. Humans may depend on innate immunity based on CRP because the pathogens involved can quickly overwhelm their host and unlike other host species their antibody against ChoP does not appear to be protective. CRP, recently noted to be present in airway surface fluid, also inhibits binding of ChoP-expressing bacteria to rPAF. The inhibitory effect of CRP on adherence of both *H. influenzae* and *S. pneumoniae* is blocked by human surfactant, an abundant component of the lower airway that is composed largely of choline phosphate and binds to CRP. The effect of surfactant could contribute to the susceptibility of the lower airway to organisms that asymptomatically colonize the upper airway where there is no surfactant. It appears, therefore, that ChoP on the cell-surface of a variety of otherwise dissimilar pathogens may be 1) important for successful colonization of the mucosal surface, and 2) evasion of innate host defenses mechanisms.

THE ROLE OF TGFSS SIGNALS DURING EMBRYOGENESIS

Malcolm Whitman, Ph.D.
Department of Cell Biology
Harvard Medical School

Our laboratory studies the mechanisms by which intercellular signals regulate the differentiation and patterning of the early vertebrate embryo. Our work is currently focused on the role of TGFß signals during embryogenesis. TGFß superfamily ligands have long been known to play essential roles in patterning at multiple steps in vertebrate embryogenesis, but, until recently, the signal transduction pathways by which TGFß factors act have been obscure. Several years ago, we discovered a novel transcription factor, FAST-1, that interacts in a ligand regulated manner with the TGFß signal transducers Smad2 and Smad4, and demonstrated that this interaction targets the Smads for specific, developmentally regulated promoters. The Smads are regulated directly by TGFß receptors, and therefore the identification of the Smad/FAST DNA binding complex provided the first example of a direct pathway by which TGFßs regulate a specific set of transcriptional responses. We have subsequently shown that FAST-1 is an essential component of the TGFß signaling pathway that establishes the early embryonic body plan.

More recently, we have used antibodies specific for the phosphorylated, activated forms of the Smads to examine how TGFß signaling is regulated endogenously during embryogenesis. We have found that the ability of embryonic cells to respond to specific TGFß ligands is regulated as development progresses, and that a small extracellular protein, cripto, acts as a specific co-receptor for one subset of TGFß ligands, the nodals, during early development. We are currently studying how cripto is regulated in the early embryo. We have also shown that nodals act via a novel mechanism, heterodimerization, to antagonize other TGFß superfamily ligands during early embryogenesis. These studies suggest that direct interactions among distantly related TGFß ligands may be important determinants of their activity in the embryo.

RO SMALL RNPS FUNCTION IN THE RECOVERY OF CELLS FROM RADIATION DAMAGE

X. Chen, H. Shi, J. Smith, D. Yang,[1] L. Evangelisti,[1] R. Flavell[1]
and Sandra Wolin, M.D., Ph.D.
Department of Cell Biology
Yale University
[1]Section of Immunobiology, HHMI, Yale University School of Medicine

The Ro 60 kDa autoantigen is an RNA-binding protein that is normally bound to small cytoplasmic RNAs known as Y RNAs. Although these RNPs are components of most vertebrate cells, their function has long been mysterious. In *Xenopus* oocyte nuclei, the Ro protein is also complexed with a large class of variant 5S rRNA precursors. Because these variant RNAs are inefficiently processed to mature 5S rRNA and eventually degraded, the Ro protein may recognize improperly folded 5S rRNA precursors as part of a quality control pathway (O'Brien and Wolin, Genes & Dev. 8:2891-2903).

Although Ro RNPs have not been detected in either *S. cerevisiae* or *S. pombe*, the genome of the radiation-resistant eubacterium *Deinococcus radiodurans* contains an orthologue of the Ro protein. The Ro protein orthologue, Rsr (Ro Sixty Related) contributes to the resistance of *D. radiodurans* to ultraviolet irradiation. *D. radiodurans* cells lacking *rsr* are more sensitive to UV irradiation than wild-type cells. During recovery from irradiation, the levels of Rsr increase approximately fourfold. Rsr binds several small RNAs, encoded upstream of *rsr*, that also accumulate during recovery from UV irradiation. Remarkably, one of these RNAs resembles the Y RNAs bound by the Ro autoantigen in higher eukaryotes (Chen et al., Genes & Dev. 14:777-82).

We have been examining the role of Ro RNPs in the recovery of higher cells following UV irradiation. Using gene knockout technology, we generated mouse embryonic stem cells that lack the Ro protein. Mouse cells lacking Ro have drastically reduced levels of Y RNAs, suggesting that Ro protein binding stabilizes these RNAs from degradation. Most interestingly, cells lacking the Ro protein are more sensitive to ultraviolet light than wild-type cells. Thus, in both mouse and bacterial cells, Ro RNPs contribute to survival following radiation damage. Although the mechanism is under investigation, one possibility is that the Ro protein binds to misfolded, mutant RNAs that are transcribed from DNA molecules containing radiation-induced mutations.

ENVIRONMENTAL RESPONSIVENESS OF THE DIMORPHIC FUNGAL PATHOGEN *HISTOPLASMA CAPSULATUM*

Jon P. Woods, M.D., Ph.D.
Department of Medical Microbiology and Immunology
University of Wisconsin, Madison

Histoplasma capsulatum (Hc) is a thermally dimorphic fungus that is a significant cause of respiratory and systemic disease in humans and other mammals. Its clinical importance has increased along with the growing immunodeficiency of the human population associated with HIV/AIDS, cancer and its treatments, immunosuppressive therapy for transplants and inflammatory syndromes, aging, and hospitalization. Hc lives saprobically in the soil as a mold, which is a successful member of a competitive polymicrobial ecosystem. The host-adapted parasitic morphotype is a budding yeast which is a facultative intracellular pathogen of macrophages. This microbe faces a variety of different environments and must survive under harsh conditions or modulate its microenvironment to achieve success as a pathogen in a professionally antimicrobial host cell. We have used several molecular techniques to identify fungal genes that are differentially expressed during infection of host macrophages and/or mice, when Hc is subjected to a complex range of environmental conditions. These methods have included in vivo expression technology (IVET), differential display, and cDNA representational difference analysis (RDA). Such approaches do not provide exhaustive genomic surveys in this eukaryotic microorganism, but we have identified several interesting genes. One differentially expressed gene encodes a small transcript in antisense orientation to a homolog of a negative regulatory protein kinase gene from another fungus, which is important in mating and starvation responses. We are examining both upstream and downstream aspects of this potential regulatory system in Hc, such as the specific environmental stimuli influencing expression of the antisense transcript, whether expression of the antisense transcript affects sense transcript expression, whether the sense transcript encodes a protein kinase functional in Hc, what the downstream targets of the putative kinase are, and the role of this locus in Hc biology and pathogenesis. A second target gene is expressed specifically in the yeast morphotype and not in mold, and the predicted encoded protein displays significant sequence homology with epidermal growth factor (EGF) domains found in a variety of proteins from other organisms, that typically function in attachment or intercellular signaling. Finally, we have preliminarily identified homologs of genes in other organisms that are involved in iron uptake. This finding interfaces with our separate interest in iron acquistion and fungal responses to the specific environmental stress of iron limitation. The essential nutrient iron lies at the competitive interface between the mammalian host and nearly all microbial pathogens, including Hc. The host displays both constitutive and inducible iron sequestration mechanisms. Iron limitation acts as an important host defense mechanism against Hc in human and mouse macrophage cell culture infection models. As a successful pathogen, Hc must express iron acquisition mechanisms to obtain this nutrient in the competitive host environment in which it resides during infection. Hc previously has been shown to produce hydroxamate siderophores, which typically act as iron-scavenging compounds. We have demonstrated ferric reduction by Hc via at least three moieties—an extracellular ferric reductase enzyme, extracellular ferric reductant(s), and cell-surface ferric reducing agent(s). Reduction of ferric to ferrous iron causes removal from both host (e.g., transferrin) and fungal (siderophore) iron-binding compounds. Siderophore-mediated and reductive processes may provide important alternate, complementary, or interactive mechanisms for acquiring iron in the soil and/or the host.

MERGING BIOLOGY WITH DRUG DISCOVERY IN OBESITY, INFLAMMATION, ANGIOGENESIS, MUSCLE DISEASE AND OTHER SETTINGS

George D. Yancopoulos M.D., Ph.D.
President, Regeneron Laboratories
Chief Scientific Officer, Regeneron Pharmaceuticals, Inc.

Growth factor and cytokines, released by one cell and acting via cell surface receptors on a second cell, mediate intercellular communications required for the initiation and/or regulation of all biologic processes. A major focus for us at Regeneron has been to identify new growth factors and/or their receptor systems, with the notion that identification of such critical master regulatory systems would present new therapeutic opportunities. We have particularly focused on growth factor/receptor systems that specifically act on a single or limited number of cell types, so that manipulation of these systems could be attempted so as to benefit diseases involving those cell types, without having widespread side effects. Over the last decade, our efforts have led to the discovery and characterization of multiple growth factor/receptor systems (e.g., neurotrophins and their Trk receptors; CNTF/IL6 family and their gp130-related receptors; agrin and its MuSK receptor; collagens and their DDR receptors; ephrins and their Eph receptors; angiopoietins and their Tie receptors;

cartilage-specific ROR receptors), as well as to novel approaches for blocking these and other growth factor systems using engineered versions of soluble receptors we term Traps.

In many cases, the growth factors or their blockers are in, or are approaching, clinical testing. I will discuss the progress of a second-generation version of CNTF, termed Axokine, which is in Phase III clinical testing for obesity, as well as Traps that we are using to block IL-1 in rheumatoid arthritis, VEGF in cancer, and IL-4 and IL-13 in asthma and allergy. I will also discuss our new high-throughput knockout and transgenic technology, termed Velocigene, which we use to rapidly assign function to genes, with examples involving genes we have realized play key roles in the biology and pathology of muscle, cartilage, blood vessels, and lymphatic vessels.

STUDIES OF 53BP1 MAY REVEAL AN UNEXPECTED LINK BETWEEN DNA DAMAGE AND MITOSIS

S.T. Liu, Y. Adachi,[1] and Tim J. Yen, Ph.D.
Fox Chase Cancer Center
[1]University of Edinburgh, Edinburgh, U.K.

53BP1 was identified as a yeast two-hybrid interactor of the p53 tumor suppressor but the functional significance of this interaction remains unclear. 53BP1 contains two copies of a BRCT motif that is found in a large number of proteins that are involved with various aspects of DNA replication, repair, and recombination. Furthermore, 53BP1 has been shown to accumulate at dozens of foci within nuclei that contain damaged DNA. Although the functionality of DNA damage induced foci remain to be clarified, it is generally believed to represent a macromolecular assembly of multiple proteins at or near the site of broken DNA. These findings strongly suggest that 53BP1 is a component of the DNA damage response pathway.

We have recently discovered that 53BP1 may have a different function besides DNA damage. 53BP1 accumulates in several large aggregates in nuclei of normal cycling cells. In mitotic cells, 53BP1 is dispersed from these aggregates and becomes concentrated at kinetochores, a structure that links chromosomes to the mitotic spindle. We determined that the earliest time that 53BP1 can be detected at kinetochores is shortly after nuclear envelope breakdown. 53BP1 assembles onto kinetochores after several other proteins that assemble onto kinetochore just prior to nuclear envelope breakdown. The temporal pattern of kinetochore binding exhibited by 53BP1 suggests that it is likely to provide functions important for the final steps of kinetochore assembly. To begin to understand the importance of 53BP1 to kinetochore function, we have localized the kinetochore targeting domain to lie within the region that contains the BRCT repeats.

Given that 53BP1 form foci of similar size at sites of DNA damage and kinetochores, we speculate that 53BP1 provides functions that are shared by these two different cellular functions. Thus, our studies of the mitotic functions of 53BP1 may provide novel insights into the mechanism by which cells monitor and respond to double stranded DNA breaks.

Appendixes

Appendix A

Agenda

LUCILLE P. MARKEY CHARITABLE TRUST SCHOLARS CONFERENCE

Friday, June 28, 2002

5:00–6:00	Welcome Party	**Adult Pool Area**

6:00–7:30   Dinner—Welcome and Introductory Remarks
            Queta Bond, Committee Chair

7:30–8:00   Bruce Alberts, President, National Academy of Sciences

8:00–10:00 Music and Socializing

Saturday, June 29, 2002

7:00–8:30	Breakfast	**Ocean Terrace**

8:30–8:40   Introduction of William Sutter   **Caribbean Ballroom**
            Lee Sechrest, Committee Member

8:40–9:00   William Sutter, Markey Trustee

9:00–9:05   Introduction of Krystyna Issacs
            George Reinhart, NAS Markey Evaluation
            Study Director

9:05–9:30	Krystyna Isaacs, *Progress of the Markey Scholars Evaluation*	

9:30–9:35   Introduction of George Yancopoulos, Markey Scholar
              Virginia Weldon, Committee Member

9:35–10:05   George Yancopoulos, Markey Scholar Presentation

10:05–10:25   Break

10:25–10:30   Introduction of Daniel Madison, Markey Scholar
              Bill Butler, Committee Member

10:30–11:00   Daniel Madison, Markey Scholar Presentation

11:00–11:05   Introduction of James Kadonaga, Markey Scholar
              Holly Smith, Committee Member

11:05–11:35   James Kadonaga, Markey Scholar Presentation

11:35–12:35	Lunch	**Salon 9**

12:35–12:40   Introduction of Gerald Rubin
              Elaine Gallin, Committee Member

12:40–1:10   Lunch Presentation
              Gerald Rubin, *The Future of Non-Profit Funding of Biomedical Research*

1:10–3:00	Poster Session I and Networking	**Ocean Terrace Foyer**

6:30–7:30	Cocktail Party	**Ocean Terrace**

7:30–8:30	Dinner	**Salon 9**

8:30–8:35   Introduction of Shirley Tilghman
              Georgine Pion, Committee Member

8:35–9:00   Dinner Presentation
              Shirley Tilghman, *Women in Science*

Sunday, June 30, 2002

7:00–8:30   Breakfast   **Ocean Terrace**

8:30–8:35   Introduction of Harold Varmus   **Caribbean Ballroom**
               James Wyngaarden, Committee Member

8:35–9:05   Harold Varmus, *New Directions in Biomedical Research*

9:05–9:10   Introduction of David Schwartz, Markey Scholar
               Mary Lou Pardue, Committee Member

9:10–9:40   David Schwartz, Markey Scholar Presentation

9:40–9:45   Introduction of Ann Stock, Markey Scholar
               Virginia Weldon, Committee Member

9:45–10:15   Ann Stock, Markey Scholar Presentation

10:15–10:35   Break

10:35–10:40   Introduction of Sandra Schmid, Markey Scholar
               Holly Smith, Committee Member

10:40–11:10   Sandra Schmid, Markey Scholar Presentation

11:10–12:30   Poster Session and Networking   **Ocean Terrace**
                                                                Foyer

12:30–1:30   Lunch   **Salon 9**

1:30–1:35   Introduction of Janet Rowley
               Georgine Pion, Committee Member

1:35–2:00   Lunch Presentation
               Janet Rowley, *New Directions in Genomic Research*

2:00   Adjourn

Appendix B

Speaker's Biographical Sketches

Krystyna Isaacs is an independent evaluation consultant in the biomedical sciences. Her clients include the National Research Council, the Howard Hughes Medical Institute (HHMI), the American Association for the Advancement of Science, and the Burroughs Wellcome Fund. Previously she was a Program Analyst at the HHMI and a staff fellow at the National Institutes of Mental Health (NIMH). Dr. Isaacs received her Ph.D. in neuroscience from the University of Illinois, Urbana-Champagne and completed a postdoc at NIMH.

James T. Kadonaga is Professor and Vice Chair of the Section of Molecular Biology, University of California, San Diego. His lab employs a primarily biochemical approach to the study of the following areas: (1) basal transcription by RNA polymerase II, (2) the role of chromatin structure in the regulation of gene expression, and (3) the mechanism of chromatin assembly. He received his Ph.D. in Chemistry from Harvard University and his postdoctoral work was done at the University of California, Berkeley in the lab of Robert Tjian.

Daniel V. Madison is a Professor in the Department of Molecular and Cell Physiology at Stanford University School of Medicine. His research focuses on the uses of electrophysiological techniques to study the mechanisms of synaptic transmission and plasticity in the mammalian hippocampus. The main focus of the lab is the study of long term potentiation (LTP) and long-term depression (LTD), the most widely studied and compelling models for the mechanisms underlying memory formation in the mammalian central nervous system. Dr. Madison received his Ph.D. in cellular biology from the University of California, San Francisco and continued his postdoctoral research there.

Janet D. Rowley is the Blum-Riese Distinguished Service Professor of Medicine at the University of Chicago Medical Center where she has spent her entire professional career. Her research focuses on the cytogenetic analysis of cells from patients with leukemia and preleukemia conditions. This analysis is performed using standard techniques as well as more sophisticated techniques such as fluorescence in situ hybridization (FISH) and spectral karyatyping (SKY), Recurring translocation breakpoints are cloned to identify the genes involved in the translocations. Cloning these breakpoints provides new tools for the more precise diagnosis of the genetic changes in leukemia cells. Dr. Rowley received her M.D. from the University of Chicago. She is a member of the National Academy of Sciences and the Institute of Medicine and is a recipient of the National Medal of Science.

Gerald M. Rubin is Vice President for Biomedical Research at the Howard Hughes Medical Institute. He is also Professor of Genetics at the University of California, Berkeley, and Adjunct Professor of Biochemistry and Biophysics at the University of California, San Francisco, School of Medicine. He has held faculty positions at Harvard Medical School and the Carnegie Institution of Washington. Rubin is known for his studies on transposable elements, for the elucidation of the molecular basis of hybrid dysgenesis and for the development of genetic transformation of Drosophila with the aid of P element vectors. He received his Ph.D. degree in molecular biology from the University of Cambridge, England. Dr. Rubin's postdoctoral work was done at Stanford University with David Hogness. Dr. Rubin is a member of the National Academy of Sciences and counts among his honors the American Chemical Society Eli Lilly Award in biological chemistry.

Sandra Louise Schmid is Professor and Chairman of the Department of Cell Biology at the Scripps Research Institute. Her research aims to identify molecules involved and to define the molecular mechanisms governing receptor-mediated endocytosis. Biochemical, molecular biological, and morphological approaches are used to elucidate the mechanisms of coat assembly, cargo recruitment and the regulation of these events by GTPases (e.g., dynamin) and kinases. She received her Ph.D. in biochemistry from Stanford University and her postdoctoral research was in the Department of Cell Biology at Yale University.

David C. Schwartz is a Professor in the Departments of Chemistry, Genetics, and the Biotechnology Center at the University of Wisconsin, Madison. Previously he had served on the faculty of Carnegie Institute of Washington and New York University. His current research is in developing optical mapping, which is a system for the construction of ordered restriction maps from individual DNA molecules. The research centers on the development of new genome analysis systems, which exploit novel macromolecular phenomena, with clear goals set to answer important biological problems. The systems are a complex mix of principles derived from computer science, biochemistry, optics, genetics, surface science and micro/nanofabrication. He received his Ph.D. in biophysical chemistry from Columbia University.

Ann Stock is a Professor in the Center for Advanced Biotechnology and Medicine, the University of Medicine and Dentistry of New Jersey–Robert Wood Johnson Medical School. She is an Associate Investigator, Howard Hughes Medical Institute. Her research focus is to understand the molecular mechanisms of receptor-mediated signal transduction. In particular, research is focused on elucidating structure/function relationships in proteins involved in information processing using a combination of molecular genetic, biochemical, and X-ray crystallographic methods. Specific interest is directed toward investigating the role of covalent modifications of proteins in signaling pathways. She received her Ph.D. in biochemistry from the University of California, Berkeley and participated in postdoctoral research at Princeton University and Brandeis University.

Shirley M. Tilghman is President of Princeton University. Before assuming the presidency, she had served as professor of molecular biology at Princeton, was a Howard Hughes Medical Institute investigator, an adjunct professor in biochemistry at the Robert Wood Johnson Medical School, and an investigator at the Institute for Cancer Research in Philadelphia. During postdoctoral studies at the National Institutes of Health, she made a number of groundbreaking discoveries while participating in cloning the first mammalian gene. She was also one of the founding members of the National Advisory Council of the Human Genome Project Initiative for the National Institutes of Health. Dr. Tilghman is renowned not only for her pioneering research, but for her national leadership on behalf of women in science and for promoting efforts to make the early careers of young scientists as meaningful and productive as possible. She received her Ph.D. in biochemistry from Temple University. Dr. Tilghman is a member of the National Academy of Sciences and the Institute of Medicine.

Harold E. Varmus is President of the Memorial Sloan-Kettering Cancer Center. He previously has served as the director of the National Institutes of Health and served on the faculty at the University of California, San Francisco where he and Dr. J. Michael Bishop and their co-workers demonstrated the cellular origins of the oncogene of a chicken retrovirus. This discovery led to the isolation of many cellular genes that normally control growth and development and are frequently mutated in human cancer. For this work, Bishop and Varmus received many awards, including the 1989 Nobel Prize for Physiology or Medicine. He is also widely recognized for his studies of the replication cycles of retroviruses and hepatitis B viruses, the functions of genes implicated in cancer, and the development of mouse models for human cancer. Dr. Varmus received his M.D. from Columbia University. He is a member of the National Academy of Sciences and the Institute of Medicine.

George D. Yancopoulos is President of Regeneron Laboratories, Inc. and Chief Scientific Officer/Senior Vice President of Research, Regeneron Pharmaceuticals, Inc. He has served on the faculty of Columbia University and New York Medical College. Dr. Yancopoulos' diverse work in the growth factor field is tied together by his continuing insights that serve to provide useful unifying models, and by his attempts to uncover therapeutically promising agents. Essentially all the discoveries of Dr. Yancopoulos and his group are moving towards the clinic—whether it be neurotrophic factors in neurological diseases and obesity, cytokine antagonists in immunologic disorders such as asthma and rheumatoid arthritis, or angiogenic regulators in cancer and vascular disease. He received both M.D. and Ph.D. degrees from Columbia University.

Appendix C

Conference Participants

Bruce Alberts
National Academy of Sciences
Washington, DC

Herman Alvarado
National Research Council
Washington, DC

Paul H. Axelson
University of Pennsylvania
Philadelphia, PA

Margaret H. Baron
Mount Sinai School of Medicine
New York, NY

Joseph M. Beechem
Molecular Probes, Inc.
Eugene, OR

Howard Benjamin
PRACEIS Pharmaceuticals
Cambridge, MA

Enriqueta C. Bond
Burroughs-Wellcome Fund
Research Triangle, NC

Stephen J. Brant
Vanderbilt University Medical
    Center
Nashville, TN

William T. Butler
Baylor College of Medicine
Houston, TX

Andrew Chisholm
University of California, Santa
    Cruz
Santa Cruz, CA

Stephen T. Crews
University of North Carolina,
    Chapel Hill
Chapel Hill, NC

Seth A. Darst
The Rockefeller University
New York, NY

Michael A. Davitz
Goldens Bridge, NY

John Dickason
Lucille P. Markey Charitable Trust
Coral Gables, FL

Jennifer A. Doudna/HHMI
Yale University School of
    Medicine
New Haven, CT

Alexander Duncan
Cambridge Antibody Technology,
    Ltd.
Cambridgeshire, UK

Geoffrey M. Duyk
Millennium Pharmaceuticals, Inc.
New Haven, CT

Joanne N. Engle
University of California, San
    Francisco
San Francisco, CA

James J. Figge
St. Peter's Hospital
Albany, NY

Simon Foote
The Walter and Eliza Hall
    Institute of Medical Research
Melbourne, AUS

Abram Gabriel
Rutgers University–CABM
Piscataway, NJ

Elaine Gallin
Doris Duke Charitable Foundation
New York, NY

Alfred L. George, Jr.
Vanderbilt University School of
    Medicine
Nashville, TN

Christopher K. Glass
University of California, San
    Diego
La Jolla, CA

Alan L. Golding
University of California, Irvine
Irvine, CA

Eric D. Greene
National Institutes of Health
Bethesda, MD

Min Han
University of Colorado at
    Boulder/HHMI
Boulder, CO

Wendy Lynn Havran
Scripps Research Institute
La Jolla, CA

Gail E. Herman
The Ohio State University
Columbus, OH

Douglas Hilton
The Walter and Eliza Hall
    Institute of Medical Research
Melbourne, AUS

David M. Hockenbery
Fred Hutchinson Cancer Research
    Center
Seattle, WA

Merl F. Hoekstra
Epoch Biosciences, Inc.
Monroe, WA

Simon Hughes
The Randall Institute, Kings'
    College
London, UK

Elizabeth Briggs Huthnance
National Research Council
Washington, DC

Krystyna Isaacs
SciConsult
Coppell, TX

Daniel G. Jay
Tufts University
Cambridge, MA

James T. Kadonaga
University of California, San
    Diego
La Jolla, CA

Chris A. Kaiser
Massachusetts Institute of
    Technology
Cambridge, MA

Lawrence C. Katz
Duke University Medical Center/
    HHMI
Durham, NC

Daniel P. Kelly
Washington University School of
    Medicine
St. Louis, MO

David M. Kingsley
Stanford University School of
    Medicine/HHMI
Stanford, CA

Stacey Kozlouski
National Research Council
Washington, DC

Mark A. Krasnow
Stanford University School of
    Medicine/HHMI
Stanford, CA

Elaine Lawson
National Research Council
Washington, DC

Peter Leedman
University of Western Australia
Perth, AUS

Michael R. Lieber
University of Southern California
    School of Medicine
Los Angeles, CA

Daniel V. Madison
Stanford University School of
    Medicine
Stanford, CA

Nigel Maidment
University of California, Los
    Angeles
Los Angeles, CA

Benjamin L. Margolis
University of Michigan Medical
   School/HHMI
Ann Arbor, MI

Malcolm Martin
National Institutes of Health
Bethesda, MD

Michael McClelland
Sidney Kimmel Cancer Center
San Diego, CA

Marcus Meister
Harvard University
Cambridge, MA

Jonathan Samuel Minden
Carnegie Mellon University
Pittsburgh, PA

John Oates
Vanderbilt University School of
   Medicine
Nashville, TN

Mary-Lou Pardue
Massachusetts Institute of
   Technology
Cambridge, MA

Andrew Perkins
Monash University
Victoria, AUS

Norbert Perrimon
Harvard Medical School/HHMI
Boston, MA

Georgine Pion
Vanderbilt University
Nashville, TN

Sharon L. Reed
University of California, San
   Diego
San Diego, CA

George R. Reinhart
National Research Council
Washington, DC

David A. Relman
Stanford University School of
   Medicine
Stanford, CA

Donald C. Rio
University of California, Berkeley
Berkeley, CA

Janet Rowley
University of Chicago
Chicago, IL

Gerald Rubin
Howard Hughes Medical Institute
Bethesda, MD

Sandra L. Schmid
The Scripps Research Institute
La Jolla, CA

David C. Schwartz
New York University
New York, NY

Lee Sechrest
University of Arizona
Tucson, AZ

Gregg L. Semenza
Johns Hopkins University School
   of Medicine
Baltimore, MD

Arlene Sharpe
Brigham and Women's Hospital
Boston, MA

George L. Shinn
Lucille P. Markey Charitable Trust
Morristown, NJ

Eric Shooter
Stanford University
Stanford, CA

Lloyd H. Smith
University of California, San
    Francisco
San Francisco, CA

Ann Stock
UMDNJ-Robert Wood Johnson
    Medical School
Piscataway, NJ

William P. Sutter
Lucille P. Markey Charitable Trust
Winnetka, IL

Shirley Tilghman
Princeton University
Princeton, NJ

Richard A. Van Etten
Harvard Medical School
Boston, MA

Harold Varmus
Dana Farber Cancer Institute
Boston, MA

David Vaux
The Walter and Eliza Hall
    Institute of Medical Research
Melbourne, AUS

Nancy Weber
Lucille P. Markey Charitable Trust
Jacksonville, FL

Jeffrey N. Weiser
University of Pennsylvania
Philadelphia, PA

Virginia Weldon
Monsanto, Company (Ret.)
St. Louis, MO

Malcolm R. Whitman
Harvard Medical School
Boston, MA

Sandra L. Wolin
Yale University School of
    Medicine
New Haven, CT

Jon P. Woods
University of Wisconsin Medical
    School
Madison, WI

James Wyngaarden
Duke University
Durham, NC

George D. Yancopoulos
Regeneron Pharmaceuticals, Inc.
Tarrytown, NY

Tim J. Yen
Fox Chase Cancer Center
Philadelphia, PA